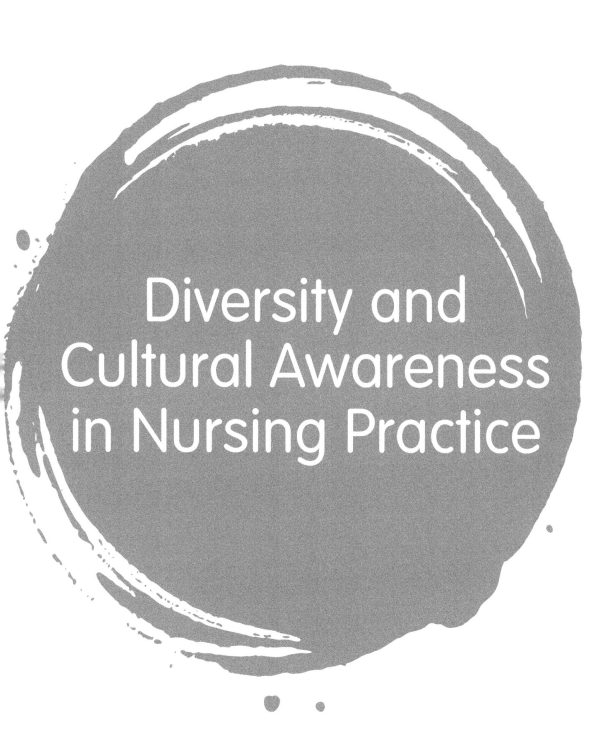

# Diversity and Cultural Awareness in Nursing Practice

Sara Miller McCune founded SAGE Publishing in 1965 to support the dissemination of usable knowledge and educate a global community. SAGE publishes more than 1000 journals and over 800 new books each year, spanning a wide range of subject areas. Our growing selection of library products includes archives, data, case studies and video. SAGE remains majority owned by our founder and after her lifetime will become owned by a charitable trust that secures the company's continued independence.

Los Angeles | London | New Delhi | Singapore | Washington DC | Melbourne

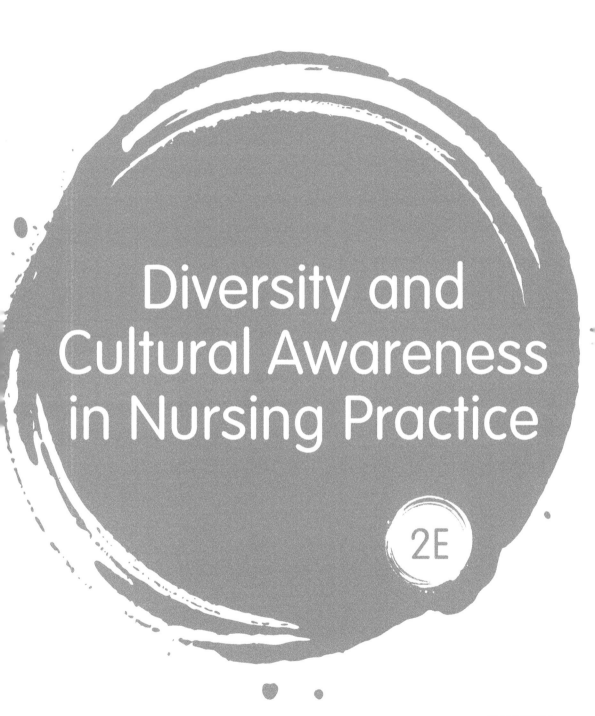

# Diversity and Cultural Awareness in Nursing Practice

2E

Edited by
Beverley Brathwaite

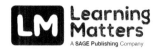

Learning Matters
A SAGE Publishing Company
1 Oliver's Yard
55 City Road
London EC1Y 1SP

SAGE Publications Inc.
2455 Teller Road
Thousand Oaks, California 91320

SAGE Publications India Pvt Ltd
B 1/I 1 Mohan Cooperative Industrial Area
Mathura Road
New Delhi 110 044

SAGE Publications Asia-Pacific Pte Ltd
3 Church Street
#10-04 Samsung Hub
Singapore 049483

Editor: Martha Cunneen
Development editor: Eleanor Rivers
Senior project editor: Chris Marke
Marketing manager: Ruslana Khatagova
Cover design: Sheila Tong
Typeset by: C&M Digitals (P) Ltd, Chennai, India

**Library of Congress Control Number:** 2023930600

**British Library Cataloguing in Publication Data**

A catalogue record for this book is available from the British Library

ISBN 978-1-5297-7926-4
ISBN 978-1-5297-7927-1 (pbk)

# Contents

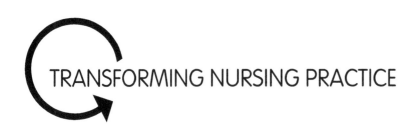

# TRANSFORMING NURSING PRACTICE

*Transforming Nursing Practice* is a series tailor made for pre-registration student nurses. Each book in the series is:

Affordable

Mapped to the NMC Standards of proficiency for registered nurses

Full of active learning features

Focused on applying theory to practice

Each book addresses a core topic and has been carefully developed to be simple to use, quick to read and written in clear language.

An invaluable series of books that explicitly relates to the NMC standards. Each book covers a different topic that students need to explore in order to develop into a qualified nurse... I would recommend this series to all Pre-Registered nursing students whatever their field or year of study.

Many titles in the series are on our recommended reading list and for good reason - the content is up to date and easy to read. These are the books that actually get used beyond training and into your nursing career.

**LINDA ROBSON,**
Senior Lecturer at Edge Hill University

**EMMA LYDON,**
Adult Student Nursing

## ABOUT THE SERIES EDITORS

**DR MOOI STANDING** is an Independent Nursing Consultant (UK and International) and is responsible for the core knowledge, adult nursing and personal and professional learning skills titles. She is an experienced NMC Quality Assurance Reviewer of educational programmes and a Professional Regulator Panellist on the NMC Practice Committee. Mooi is also Board member of Special Olympics Malaysia, enabling people with intellectual disabilities to participate in sports and athletics nationally and internationally.

**DR SANDRA WALKER** is a Clinical Academic in Mental Health working between Southern Health Trust and the University of Southampton and responsible for the mental health nursing titles. She is a Qualified Mental Health Nurse with a wide range of clinical experience spanning more than 25 years.

# BESTSELLING TEXTBOOKS

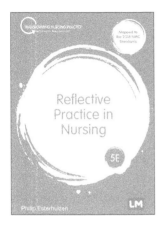

Reflective Practice in Nursing
5E
Philip Esterhuizen
LM

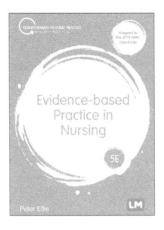

Evidence-based Practice in Nursing
5E
Peter Ellis
LM

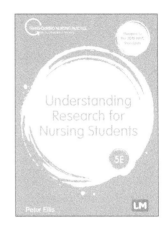

Understanding Research for Nursing Students
5E
Peter Ellis
LM

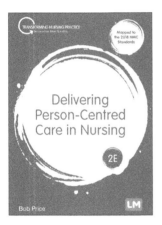

Delivering Person-Centred Care in Nursing
2E
Bob Price
LM

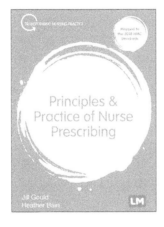

Principles & Practice of Nurse Prescribing
Jill Gould
Heather Bain
LM

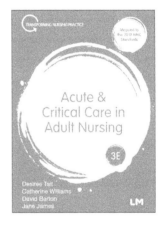

Acute & Critical Care in Adult Nursing
3E
Desiree Tait
Catherine Williams
David Barton
Jane James
LM

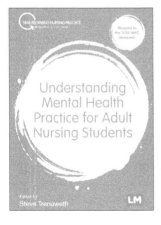

Understanding Mental Health Practice for Adult Nursing Students
Edited by
Steve Trenoweth
LM

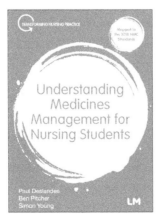

Understanding Medicines Management for Nursing Students
Paul Deslandes
Ben Pitcher
Simon Young
LM

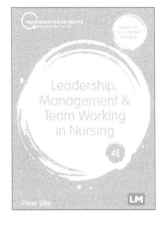

Leadership, Management & Team Working in Nursing
4E
Peter Ellis
LM

You can find a full list of textbooks in the *Transforming Nursing Practice* series at

## https://uk.sagepub.com/TNP-series

# About the authors

**Beverley Brathwaite** is a registered adult nurse, who worked clinically in acute general medicine, tissue viability, practice development, and telephone triage. Beverley is a registered teacher with the Nursing and Midwifery Council (NMC), senior fellow with the higher education academy (SFHEA) nearing completion of her PhD, and a senior lecturer at the University of Roehampton. Beverley's teaching focus has ranged from tissue viability to acute and long-term nursing care, evidence-based practice, to inequalities in health and diversity. She has worked with undergraduate and postgraduate degree students from all fields, as well as nursing associates. She has written journal articles and book chapters and presented at national and international conferences on Black British nurses' professional experiences, COVID-19 and minority infections rates, the awarding gap of Black and Brown student nurses, and racism in nursing and the NHS.

**Gillian Craig** PhD is an independent consultant who specialises in public health and social science, with a particular interest in social diversity and inclusion in health. Her research areas include psychosocial models of practice for those experiencing tuberculosis. She has developed guidance on providing psychosocial counselling and adherence support and has co-authored several chapters in the *Tuberculosis Stigma Measurement Guidance* developed by the USAID-funded, KNCV-led Challenge TB project.

**Caroline McGraw** PhD registered as an adult general nurse in 1991. She has been working in district nursing practice for over 15 years and completed her primary healthcare nursing PGDip (district nurse) with specialist practitioner qualification in 2003. She is a registered teacher with the NMC, and a SFHEA. Her key interest at the doctoral level was in applying conceptual models developed to predict risk and analyse adverse events in secondary care environments to the domiciliary care setting. Her key research interests include medication management with older people living at home, the interface between health and social care in the community, and risk management in domiciliary care settings. Her current practice involves palliative care in hospice settings.

**Mariama Seray-Wurie** is head of practice learning at the University of Roehampton, where she is responsible for the strategic and operational oversight of practice learning, ensuring effective practice learning processes for the nursing programme that meet university and regulatory body requirements. She became a registered nurse in 1989 and her clinical background was in infectious diseases and haematology before moving to higher education in 2000, starting her career in nurse education as a clinical skills facilitator. Mariama has been a lecturer at the University of West London, a senior lecturer for adult nursing and a director of programmes at Middlesex University. She graduated with an MA in Learning and Teaching in Healthcare in 2005 and her teaching focus is mainly on pre-registration nursing curriculum development and programme management, simulated practice learning, and international exchanges in nursing.

**Marion Hinds** is a senior lecturer in adult nursing at Middlesex University with over 37 years of clinical nursing experience in intensive and high-dependency nursing. She has an MA in policy organisation and change in professional care and is a registered teacher with the NMC. Academic experience includes lecturing on pre-registration and post-registration programmes. She has a particular interest in the theory and practice of the nursing process and care planning and is co-chair of a biannual care planning conference for nursing students. Marion has also presented at national and international conferences.

**Nicky Lambert** is an associate professor (practice) at Middlesex University, where she is director of teaching and learning for mental health, social work, and integrative medicine. She is registered as a specialist practitioner (NMC) and is a SFHEA. Nicky has worked across a range of mental health services both in the UK and internationally, supporting staff and practice development in acute and mental health trusts, councils, businesses, and charities. She is also a specialist advisor on women's well-being, mental health, and nurse education. She is a community activist, a researcher, and a trustee for a women's centre.

# Introduction

*Beverley Brathwaite*

# Who is this book for?

This book is aimed at undergraduate pre-registration nursing students and nursing associates who will complete their programmes and register with the Nursing and Midwifery Council (NMC). The NMC has clearly identified the importance of student nurses being able to deliver care to diverse patient groups.

# The role of the nurse in the twenty-first century

Registered nurses provide leadership in the delivery of care for people of all ages, physical and emotional abilities, genders, and from different ethnicities and cultural backgrounds. They provide nursing care for people who have complex mental, physical, cognitive, and behavioural care needs, those living with dementia, the elderly, and for people at the end of their life (NMC, 2018a, p3).

The main areas of this book cover generic aspects of the knowledge, skills, and attributes that are vital to learning about healthcare from a diversity and cultural perspective. These skills and attributes will be valuable to students of all fields of nursing and midwifery. The NMC Standards of Proficiency for Registered Nurses (NMC, 2018a) is the framework on which the book is based. As with all the titles in the Transforming Nursing Practice series, the content of this book is useful for anyone who is studying to become a healthcare professional.

# Why *Diversity and Cultural Awareness in Nursing Practice?*

Since the last edition of the book, the world has changed dramatically in relation to health. COVID-19 has had a dramatic impact on health and social care. Nurses from all fields have been at the forefront of what has been called the battle against COVID-19 and the impact it has had on human life. Nationally and internationally COVID-19 has affected the delivery of care, highlighting inequalities in access to health, health outcomes, and the organisation of care. The diverse members of populations have had varied experiences of healthcare due to COVID-19 and some of these issues will be addressed.

Our patients are individual members of society who are living longer, meaning a larger older population. They can come from diverse ethnic, cultural, and religious backgrounds from all over the world. Their reasons for being in the UK are equally diverse, whether they are searching for a better quality of life and financial security, or escaping from war, terrorism, and fear of persecution in their homeland. Patients/service users bring their ethnicities and personal cultural and religious beliefs and customs with them. It must be remembered that throughout history, British society has been, and continues to be, heavily influenced by these cultures, religions, and ethnicities.

Members of these groups can be marginalised from society because of their differences from the majority of the population in the UK. There are other groups that can also be marginalised, such as the lesbian, gay, bisexual, trans, intersex, queer, or questioning (LGBTQIA+) community. Within this community terminology and understanding of membership is changing. Disorder of sex development (DSD) is preferred rather than intersex as it is a less derogatory term. DSD acknowledges the diversity in relation to varied chromosome pattern, reproductive gland and cells and multiple genotype and phenotype presentations (Babbar et al, 2020). Queer also has a negative and discriminatory relationship with identity as it is used as an slur but also in some parts of the gay community there is an attempt to reclaim it more positively (Corner , 2019). The book at present will continue to use the acronym LGBTQAI+ but acknowledges the complexities of meaning within its community and how it is generally used.

Other groups are those with mental health issues, physical disabilities, Gypsy Roma Travellers and the neurodiverse. The focus within the book will be learning disabilities and autism. Acknowledging that neurodiversity 'describes the idea that people experience and interact with the world around them in many different ways; there is no one "right" way of thinking, learning, and behaving, and differences are not viewed as deficits' (Harvard health Publishing 2021).

## Book structure

Chapter 1 defines the terminology and concepts that are fundamental to using this book and working with the diversity of patients who we meet as healthcare professionals. Health and inequality and equity will be examined, which will provide insight into the attitudes often held by healthcare professionals when it comes to diverse communities and care delivery.

Chapter 2 presents a broader social perspective on certain diverse groups, addressing racism, bias phobias, and stigma, considering what these continue to mean for the health of people in these groups and the delivery of care within an ever-changing population and the NHS. Concepts of social and health determinants will be expanded upon, as well as an explanation of behaviour towards access, treatment, and the attitudes of diverse communities to health and healthcare professionals.

Chapter 3 considers the crucial role of good communication in all its forms for providing effective care and ensuring good access to care for diverse groups. The evidence that defines and supports the rise in the importance of health literacy will be examined and related to the impact that poor health literacy can have on health and illness. Effective communication is the cornerstone of patient care for all fields of nursing and healthcare professionals and students. It is one of the ways in which compassion and sensitivity can be conveyed to promote collaboration and cooperation in the clinical setting. It is crucial when working with all patients including diverse patient groups.

Chapter 4 argues that an understanding of the concepts of cultural competency in relation to nursing practice is a prerequisite to the delivery of appropriate, effective, and holistic nursing care. Before the notion of cultural competency can be understood, culture and competency must be understood as separate terms. This chapter critically discusses these two concepts. The key elements of cultural competence (awareness, sensitivity, attitudes, knowledge, and skills) are then examined. Following on from this, the varied theories of cultural concepts are discussed and analysed. This will allow students to understand the complex nature of cultural competency.

A significant part of the nurse's role involves the assessment and implementation of care for patients/clients, which can occur in a variety of healthcare settings. Chapter 5 explores the role of supporting and working with individuals and families from a diverse range of backgrounds, religions, cultures, ethnicities, and disabilities, as well as from the lesbian, gay, bisexual, trans/transexual/transgender, queer/questioning, intersex, asexual (LGBTQIA+) community, which can influence how the individual perceives health and illness and how they may want to receive care.

Chapter 6 considers the definitions and theories of spirituality within diverse groups and how the nurse/student can assess the spirituality of patients in order to care for this 'hidden' need. The chapter will also show the reader how to manage their own beliefs of spirituality within the patient–nurse relationship and manage situations where their beliefs contrast with those of their patients. Healthcare professionals deal with death, grief, and loss (DGL). Diverse groups approach DGL in differing ways based on cultural and religious beliefs. Identifying needs through these differing approaches should allow culturally and religiously sensitive support to be given when delivering nursing care.

Chapter 7 offers nurses an understanding of how to address the public health needs of Britain's diverse populations in the community/primary care setting. The chapter charts the transition from communicable to non-communicable diseases, using epidemiological data, and in the light of COVID-19, highlights the ongoing threats to diverse communities that were disproportionately impacted by the pandemic. It will begin with an examination of the national public health policy background and illustrates how public health interventions, although necessary, can have unintended consequences for diverse populations because of their unique needs. It introduces the Nuffield intervention ladder, an ethical framework, to assist healthcare professionals and policymakers with making judgements about public health interventions and their impact on communities. It offers useful advice on how nurses can advocate for communities by influencing policy.

Chapter 8 argues that mental health issues are as important as physical health issues. Healthcare is delivered within a societal framework, and it is important for us to understand the ways that best mental health practices can improve patients' lives. By appreciating these issues, particularly following the onset of the pandemic, we can explore ways for all healthcare professionals to work together and engage in delivering the best care possible for mental health service users from minoritised groups.

# Requirements for the NMC Standards of Proficiency for Registered Nurses and the proficiencies and platforms

The NMC has established standards of proficiencies of practice to be met by applicants to different parts of the register, and these are the standards it considers necessary for safe and effective practice. In addition to the standards, the NMC has set out specific proficiencies that nursing students must be able to perform at various points of an education programme. These are known as 'platforms'. This book is structured so that it will help you to understand and meet the standards and proficiencies required for entry to the NMC register. The relevant proficiencies and platforms are presented at the start of each chapter so that you can clearly see which ones the chapter addresses. There are *generic standards* that all nursing students, irrespective of their field, must achieve, and *field-specific standards* relating to each field of nursing (i.e. mental health, children's, learning disability and adult nursing).

This book includes the latest standards of proficiency for registered nursing (NMC, 2018a).

# Learning features

Learning by reading text is not always easy. Therefore, to provide variety and to assist with the development of independent learning skills and the application of theory to practice, this book contains activities, case studies, scenarios, further reading, useful websites, and other materials to enable you to participate in your own learning. You will need to develop your own study skills and 'learn how to learn' to get the best from the material. The book cannot provide all the answers, but instead provides a framework for your learning.

The activities in the book in particular will help you to make sense of, and learn about, the material being presented. Some activities ask you to reflect on aspects of practice, or your experience of it, or the people or situations you encounter. *Reflection* is an essential skill in nursing, and it helps you to understand the world around you and often to identify how things might be improved. Other activities will help you to develop key graduate skills, such as your ability to *think critically* about a topic in order to challenge received wisdom, or your ability to *research a topic and find appropriate information and evidence*, and to be able to *make decisions* using that evidence in situations that are often difficult and time-pressured. Communication and working as part of a team are core to all nursing practice, and some activities will ask you to carry out *teamwork activities* or think about your *communication skills* to help develop these. Finally, as a registered nurse, you will be expected to *lead and manage* your own team, caseload or area of care, and so some activities focus on helping you build confidence in doing this.

All the activities require you to take a break from reading the text, think through the issues presented, and carry out some independent study, possibly using the internet. Where appropriate, there are sample answers presented at the end of each chapter, and these will help you to understand more fully your own reflections and independent study. Remember, academic study will always require independent work; attending lectures will never be enough to be successful in your programme, and these activities will help to deepen your knowledge and understanding of the issues under scrutiny and give you practice at working on your own.

You might want to think about completing these activities as part of your personal development plan (PDP) or portfolio. After completing an activity, write it up in your PDP or portfolio in a section devoted to that particular platform, then look back over time to see how far you are developing. You can also do more of the activities for a key skill in which you have identified a weakness, which will help build your skill and confidence in this area.

This book covers some challenging areas of society, such as racism, transphobia, discrimination, stereotyping and inequalities in health, and more recently how the COVID-19 pandemic has exacerbated some of these issues in relation to care delivery, experience, and health disparities, while considering how influential these issues are in giving holistic care to all patients. We hope that the book allows you to think not only about how you give care, but to whom, and the social context in which our patients live and healthcare delivery takes place.

# Chapter 1 Diversity, health inequality, and nursing

*Beverley Brathwaite*

## NMC Future Nurse: Standards of Proficiency for Registered Nurses

This chapter will address the following platforms and proficiencies:

**Platform 1: Being an accountable professional**

1.14  provide and promote non-discriminatory, person-centred and sensitive care at all times, reflecting on people's values and beliefs, diverse backgrounds, cultural characteristics, language requirements, needs and preferences, taking account of any need for adjustments.

**Platform 2: Promoting health and preventing ill health**

2.3  understand the factors that may lead to inequalities in health outcomes.

**Platform 7: Coordinating care**

7.9  facilitate equitable access to healthcare for people who are vulnerable or have a disability, demonstrate the ability to advocate on their behalf when required, and make necessary reasonable adjustments to the assessment, planning and delivery of their care.

## Chapter aims

After reading this chapter, you will be able to:

- understand the definitions of key terms used in the book;
- have an awareness of the multiple causes of inequality in healthcare within a diverse context;
- know the difference between equity and equality; and
- consider the difference between equity and equality and how this affects healthcare practice, as well as what to consider as a student nurse in order to make unbiased clinical decisions.

# Introduction

## Case study: Cunningham Street

In many streets in the UK, people of differing ethnicities, faiths, religions, and sexualities are living out their lives. At number 35 Cunningham Street, Anish is of Asian descent. He has type 2 diabetes and chronic kidney disease and had been shielding due to COVID-19; today he is going to see his GP. At number 12, Karen is worried about her wife having postnatal depression since the birth of their second baby six months ago in lockdown and has had an online conversation about this with the health visitor. At number 2, Olufunke is of Nigerian descent and has just recently been discharged from hospital following an admission due to her systemic lupus erythematosus (SLE). At number 5, Jennifer is a young woman of Caribbean descent who is on the autistic spectrum and is waiting for an ambulance to take her to hospital with a suspected fractured ankle. She is worried about catching COVID-19.

All the residents on Cunningham Street have come into contact with the NHS and healthcare professionals. They expect and deserve to be treated with an awareness and understanding of their particular needs and the world in which they live. As healthcare professionals, we must acknowledge that these persons encounter us as healthcare professionals in conjunction with an illness, disease, or trauma that may be acute, long-term, physical, or emotional, and it is our responsibility to respond to this professionally and holistically. The six Cs of care, compassion, competence, communication, courage, and commitment (NHS England, 2015) – as well as a seventh C, consistency, to assure that the six Cs are performed with every healthcare encounter – are an essential part of assuring that care delivery meets the requirements of patients. Acknowledging the unique differences of all patients who come from our diverse patient population is valuable in delivering high-quality care.

In this chapter, we look at diversity and 'inequality challenges', and how important it is that you understand the inequalities and social determinants of health so that equitable and individualised care can be given. It demonstrates how issues of diversity are a key component of health inequality and they must be considered carefully when planning equitable service provision. Data from the Office for National Statistics (ONS) is used to illustrate how the population has become more diverse, as well as highlighting vulnerable groups in society and in healthcare.

This chapter will show how diversity has changed in modern Britain. It will take a more detailed look at race, ethnicity, and culture, the Black Lives Matter movement, and health, and consider the importance of prejudice, stereotyping, racism, difference, and unconscious bias in relation to healthcare delivery. It will also think about the inequality this promotes and how equity and equality differ. Finally, intersectionality as a concept within health, as well as its importance in acknowledging that our patients can be treated unfairly based on multiple diverse group memberships, is also discussed.

There are a number of terms, such as ethnicity, culture, and stereotyping, that will be used throughout the book. Although we hear and use some of these terms all the time, we do not always appreciate the complexities of their meanings. The terms in this section can only be briefly defined here. Please see the further reading section at the end of the chapter for guidance on exploring these terms in more depth.

# Diversity

Diversity within the context of this book refers to the multiple points of view and experiences which can be defined by the protected characteristics of the Equality Act (2010). It can also be defined as making sure that *we recognise, respect, value and celebrate the differences that everyone has, as well as leveraging the opportunities that different people bring to the work that we do* (Health Education England, 2018, p8). These differences can be seen through the inhabitants of our street in the above case study. They can be based on ethnicity, sexual orientation, mental health issues, or learning disabilities. This shows just how multifaceted and complex diversity is. Indeed, these differences or categories are only a few of many. Others include asylum seeker, immigrant, age, and lesbian, gay, bisexual, trans/transsexual/transgender, queer/questioning, intersex, asexual (LGBTQIA+), and are just that – categories – our patients are not 'simply' categories or groups, not forgetting that an individual can identify themselves across multiple categories. Super-diversity can be understood as a lens to describe an exceptional demographic situation characterised by the multiplication of social categories within specific localities (Wessendorf, 2014).

Diversity is often characterised negatively by the media and parts of society, particularly when referring to topics surrounding ethnicity, immigration, asylum seekers, and refugees (Wessendorf, 2014). Riots have erupted because of disadvantages and inequality faced by some Black, Asian, and Minority Ethnic (BAME) groups and religious and cultural groups within some sectors of society, such as education, the criminal justice system, and healthcare (EHRC, 2016b). The term BAME is even being reconsidered as it doesn't reflect the changes that are necessary, particularly over time with how these communities want to be identified (MacInnes, 2020). Therefore, in this book the term Black and Brown (B&B) will be used to not only distinguish skin colour but identify the country of birth and descendants of Africa, the Caribbean and South Asia.

## Black Lives Matter

First, Black Lives Matter (BLM) as a movement does not mean that non-Black lives do not matter. It is a movement to end racism and gain equal and equitable treatment in society for Black people (acknowledging other racialised people of Asian, South Asian, and South American heritage). It may have started in the USA and gained more ground after the murder in May 2020 of George Floyd, an African American man, by a white police officer. It reminds mainstream society here in Britain of racism, both individual and structural, that exists and the reasons and causes of this racism; how Britain has a long history and connection to racism, particularly of B&B people; and how in healthcare it manifests itself in poorer outcomes and experiences for B&B patients. COVID-19 highlighted these poorer outcomes for B&B people and will be discussed in more detail in Chapter 2.

# Race, ethnicity, and culture

Race, ethnicity and culture are terms commonly used in healthcare literature, society, and clinical practice. These terms will be recurring throughout the book and, like diversity, are complex concepts with social, political, ideological, and sociological differences in meanings and emphases.

The term 'race' generally refers to a social group or person appearing to have observable differing characteristics, such as skin colour, facial features, and body shapes (Garner, 2017). This is breaking down multiple theories of race to their most simplistic form. However, when talking about race, it is never a simple task:

- *'Race' in biological terms (of simply what people look like) matters a lot. For example, it bears importantly on the way resources are made more or less accessible.*
- *It is not individuals alone, but also important institutions like the State, who have input in determining the meaning of 'race'.*
- *Different social systems and their cultures attach different types of meaning to physical appearance.*

(Garner, 2017, p5)

The most important aspect about 'race' to acknowledge is that it does not in fact exist. 'Race' is completely socially constructed and the concept of the inequality of specific groups based on skin colour is something that has been used over centuries to justify treating people differently. Of course, the term is used frequently, but this crucial point of social construction should be remembered.

Ethnicity refers to the importance of a collective culture that is integral to being a member of a social group and a person in this group. The focus is less on the physical attributes connected to race, but on the social grounds of shared traditions and heritage (Murji and Solomos, 2015). It is a preferred term to use as it acknowledges the social nature of being in a social group and that skin colour is not the only characteristic that can unite a group.

Tabassum (2022) defines culture in two ways. First, the values, beliefs, symbols, and language, which he calls non-material cultures. Material cultures are the second type encompassing physical objects such as tools, technology, clothing, eating utensils, and means of transportation. Whether it is values of objects, culture is the shared experiences of a group of people that connects them, and these experiences are a part of what makes the patient you are nursing who they are. To deliver effective care, healthcare professionals need to understand the cultural attachments of our patients, to friends, family, and other members of the wider community that share both ethnicity and culture.

As can be seen here, there are overlapping ideas of what 'race', ethnicity, and culture mean, and this is a theoretical and political debate that carries on today (Murji and Solomos, 2015). An important point to consider is that these are terms that are used to signify differences within society from the biggest ethnic group in England and Wales, which is white British (ONS, 2019a). Difference manifests itself within healthcare as inequality experienced by 'other' groups and the detrimental effects this has on their lives. The government has acknowledged these 'other' groups and the inequality that they experience not only within healthcare, but within society as a whole. The Equality Act 2010 brought together previous legislation, such as the Equal Pay Act 1970 and the Employment Equality (Age) Regulations 2006, under one Act of Parliament (HM Government, 2013). The Act identified the following protected characteristics: age, disability, gender reassignment, race, religion or belief (including lack of belief), sex, and sexual orientation. These groups will be discussed throughout the book. It is interesting to note that this legislation uses the terms 'sex' and 'race', not 'gender' and 'ethnicity'. This creates even more blurred lines of meaning. This is something that, as nurses/midwives, you will have to grapple with on a daily basis as your patients' identities are wrapped up in these socially constructed categories.

# Prejudice and stereotyping

In defining these two terms together, it is important to appreciate that they are inextricably linked to 'race', ethnicity, and cultural differences, leading in some cases to racism-based inequality in society, and therefore healthcare and healthcare systems. These are complex terms that have theoretically changed over time. Nelson (2015), a social psychologist, identifies prejudice as the negative attitude towards a group or towards a member of that group, and stereotyping as the traits that come to mind when we think of a group or an individual from that group that is different from another group. These differences can be based on ethnicity, religion, sexual orientation, and physical or mental abilities. There does not need to be an unequal power relationship for prejudice and stereotyping to be used by any group (Dovidio et al., 2010). However, they are inextricably linked to racism and racial discrimination, Islamophobia, antisemitism, homophobia, and transphobia. This is where the importance of power plays a vital part in how the negative traits attributed to the formation of stereotypes of particular groups lead to prejudice and then racism (or Islamophobia or antisemitism). If one group, white, Christian, historically has more power based on slavery and colonisation over 'other' groups (e.g. B&B and Gypsy, Roma, Traveller (GRT) people), then the social construct of race leading to racism becomes a part of how people interact with each other in society. This includes healthcare because people from society work and practise in healthcare. You bring these social constructs with you.

# Racism and racial discrimination

There are many theories of racism that address the concept from a historical, sociological, political, legal, and cultural perspective. Fredrickson (2015, p19–28) picks up one of the main themes highlighted in this book, which is difference. Racism has a unique power relationship that is distinct from other forms of difference and discrimination. Racial discrimination is often used interchangeably with racism. Solomos (2003) conceptualises that racial discrimination has three components: acts, processes, and practice. There is someone responsible for acting in a racially discriminative manner and there are processes that are 'established, routine and subtle' (p77) within healthcare services. These acts of racial discrimination can be perpetrated by healthcare professionals and the systems in which healthcare is delivered and do have a significant impact on patient care, well-being, and outcomes.

Within healthcare, the issue of difference and discrimination is not only racially based, but also happens to other socially disadvantaged groups, such as patients with learning disabilities, mental health problems, or belonging to the LGBTQIA+ community. However they are different, they become the 'them' to the 'normal' us, which tends to be white, heterosexual, and Christian. This allows us, as healthcare professionals, to treat 'different' patients from these groups in a way in which we would not treat others and ourselves.

# Difference, diversity, and inequality in health

Professor Lorraine Culley has written extensively on diverse groups' interactions and inequality within healthcare:

> *While these are highly disparate groups (and internally very heterogeneous), they share at least one important feature which each contribution ably demonstrates: their health is intimately bound up with the multi-faceted disadvantage that derives from the social, political and economic make-up of our society and our response to 'difference'.*

> (Culley, 2010, p299)

There are three issues here. Diverse groups have similarities, but this does not mean that each member of the group is the same and each person should be treated as an individual. These individuals and groups do not exist in a vacuum outside of societal external influences, such as class and income. As healthcare professionals, we must constantly challenge the idea that 'difference' can be reduced to people being simply unequal to the rest of 'normal' society. An acknowledgement of the intricacies of diversity and difference is important in allowing nurses to treat the patient, not the difference as to which society labels people. The BLM movement strives to highlight those ethnicities that are not white, are seen as different and are treated unequally.

Activity 1.1 asks you to consider how ethnic diversity might affect you as a healthcare professional, and how this might affect how you interact and organise your care for a patient.

## Activity 1.1   Reflection

Think about an occasion in the clinical environment that you have witnessed in which you or the patient/service user was considered to be related to ethnicity in a negative way. How did it affect the care that you or your colleagues provided?

Why do you think it is important to be aware of these issues?

*Although this activity is based on your own reflection, there is also a model answer provided at the end of the chapter.*

Having considered how an awareness of the negative issues surrounding ethnic diversity might inform your practice, we now turn to *equity* and *equality*.

# Equity and equality: are they the same?

There is a frequent misunderstanding that equity and equality are the same, and they are regularly used interchangeably, particularly when discussing health. The NHS principles are based both on equity and equality. Access to healthcare at the point of use regardless of ability to pay is the cornerstone of the NHS (National Health Service Act, 1946). Equity is accepting that equal access does not mean equitable outcomes as many diverse groups have unequitable access, treatment, and outcomes that are in part or wholly based on diversity, and the marginalisation and discrimination that comes with it. For example, the LGBTQIA+ community has experience of marginalisation and, when older (over 50), age is an added factor (Williams, 2021; Benbow and Kingston, 2022). In general, hospital patients with learning disabilities have been treated differently, which has led to death (NHS England and NHS Improvement, 2019). Racial discrimination against B&B patients has led to poorer outcomes and experiences of healthcare (Danso and Danso, 2021). The key is that in society and health, all people do not start from the same position, and if diverse groups 'lag behind' from the beginning then more time or resources are needed to assure equity. When delivering care, this is something that you should consider. It is so important that the World Health Organization states:

*Health inequities are avoidable inequalities in health between groups of people within countries and between countries. These inequities arise from inequalities within and between societies.*

(WHO, 2008c, p1)

Once an acknowledgement of inequity in health has been established, we must then look at the possible reasons for this and the terminology that is used to describe it, both globally and here at home in the UK. Below are some areas and terminology to consider.

# Black Lives Matter and health

The murder of a Black man named George Floyd on the streets of America reignited a movement that is built on the major issues of highlighting the social injustices that impact on the lives of B&B people and putting forward anti-racist strategies (Thelwall and Thelwall, 2021). Black Lives Matter (BLM) represents positive action towards equality and inclusivity. The BLM protests reminded society that racism, racial stereotypes, and racially based unconscious bias still exist not only throughout the world but in the organisations and institutions of societies. The NHS and healthcare, which are significant parts of society, are sites of inequality and unequity and we have already discussed the differences between the two and how this can influence health outcomes for B&B people, particularly when B&B people live in predominantly white societies such as England and America.

# What are the social 'determinants' of health?

*The social determinants of health are the circumstances in which people are born, grow up, live, work and age, and the systems put in place to deal with illness. These circumstances are in turn shaped by a wider set of forces: economics, social policies, and politics.*

(WHO, 2008c)

# What are the drivers of health inequalities?

*The global context affects how societies prosper through its impact on international relations and domestic norms and policies. These in turn shape the way that society, both at the national and local level, organises its affairs, giving rise to forms of social position and hierarchy, whereby populations are organised according to income, education, occupation, gender, race/ethnicity and other factors. Where people are in the social hierarchy affects the conditions in which they grow, learn, live, work and age, their vulnerability to ill health, and the consequences of ill health.*

(WHO, 2008c)

# Marmot Review: *Fair Society, Healthy Lives* (2015)

*Focusing solely on the most disadvantaged will not reduce health inequalities sufficiently. To reduce the steepness of the social gradient in health, actions must be universal, but with a scale and intensity that is proportionate to the level of disadvantage. We call this proportionate universalism.*

(Marmot et al., 2010)

The WHO and Marmot reviews (Marmot 2015; Marmot et al., 2010; Marmot et al., 2020a; Marmot et al., 2020b; Marmot et al., 2020c; Marmot et al., 2021) have been highlighted among an ongoing and growing body of evidence on the issue of social determinants. Note the similarities between these reports. It is because of this similarity nationally and internationally that they have been used. The social determinants of health are linked to diverse groups. There is also a clear relationship between the social position of our patients and how this must be considered when managing patient care in conjunction with the patient. In Chapter 2, the Marmot Review update of this report and its link to COVID-19 and B&B lives will be explored in more detail.

Activity 1.2 specifically identifies that health inequalities exist for certain ethnic groups in British society, and what, if anything, can and should be done to redress this.

## Activity 1.2  Evidence-based practice and research

Locate the National Institute for Health and Care Excellence's (NICE) Promoting health and preventing ill health and premature death in BAME groups:

www.nice.org.uk/guidance/qs167

Read through the document and find the six quality statements that are there to help local areas focus on the specific needs of the ethnic groups, disadvantaged, and excluded groups in their locality, and who uses or should be using health and social care. Consider whether you knew that there was a difference in the increased risk of type 2 diabetes. Also, the different areas of focus (statements) should make you think about how you provide care based on evidence and how the patient should be central to the use of evidence. If you are practising in an area with a high non-white population, information such as this must be something that you seek out. Ensure that you have the right information for the population in which you practise.

*An outline of what you need to consider is given at the end of the chapter.*

# Diversity: statistical data and research findings

There is much statistical data on the diversity of the UK population, policy findings, and research on diversity and health. The following are significant and provide context to the patients you will encounter in practice:

- The population of the UK in mid-2020 was estimated to be 67,026,292 (ONS, 2022b).
- In the 2011 census, 58,000 people identified themselves as Gypsy or Irish Traveller (0.1 per cent of the usual resident population of England and Wales), but it is

estimated that between 100,000–300,000 Gypsy/Travellers and up to 200,000 Roma people live in the UK (Parliament UK, 2019).
- There are 14.1 million disabled people in the UK: 8 per cent of children; 19 per cent of working age adults; 46 per cent of old age pensioners (Scope, 2021).
- There are almost 11 million people aged 65 and over – 19 per cent of the total population. In ten years, this will have increased to almost 13 million people or 22 per cent of the population (Centre for Aging Better, 2022).
- The proportion of the UK population aged 16 years and over identifying as heterosexual or straight decreased from 94.6 per cent in 2018 to 93.7 per cent in 2019. Between 2018 and 2019, the proportion of people who identified as LGB increased for England (2.7 per cent, up from 2.3 per cent) and Scotland (2.7 per cent, up from 2.0 per cent), however, Wales (2.9 per cent) and Northern Ireland (1.3 per cent) remained stable; among English regions, people in London were most likely to identify as LGB (3.8 per cent, an increase from 2.8 per cent) (ONS, 2021b).
- It is estimated that in the UK in 2022 there were 1.5 million people with learning disabilities; 1.2 million in England (Mencap, 2022).

The Equality and Human Rights Commission (EHRC, 2016a) has found the following:

- Among lesbian and bisexual women, 50 per cent of them have had negative experiences with the NHS.
- People with mental health problems have much higher rates of physical illness, with a range of factors contributing to greater prevalence of, and premature mortality from, coronary heart disease, stroke, diabetes, infections, and respiratory disease.
- People with severe mental illness die, on average, 20 years younger than the general population, often from preventable physical illnesses.
- While the UK's white population has remained roughly the same size over the past ten years, the ethnic minority population has almost doubled, and now is at least 8 million people, or 14 per cent of the UK population.
- The proportion of UK citizens from ethnic minority communities is expected to double in the next decades and will be between 20 and 30 per cent by 2050.

Furthermore:

- Gypsy, Roma, and Traveller communities may have difficulty understanding and navigating the system; had past experiences of being turned away from services and being badly treated; may be unable to speak the language or be able to read or write; and afraid of punitive action after accessing services (UK Parliament, 2019).
- Gaps remain in how reasonable adjustments are provided for disabled people accessing hospital care. It is important for hospital staff to listen to the perspectives of disabled people about the provision of reasonable adjustments and make improvements as necessary (Read et al., 2018, p8).

- People with learning disabilities die, on average, 15–20 years sooner than people in the general population, with some of these deaths identified as being potentially amenable to good-quality healthcare (University of Bristol, 2018, p5).
- Mencap (2013) notes the following in relation to those with learning disabilities in acute hospitals:

*Our cases show that, despite some encouraging evidence of a better understanding of the concept of reasonable adjustments across the NHS, a lack of compliance with the Disability Discrimination Act (now the Equality Act) underpins the failures identified by families. They illustrate both direct discrimination from NHS staff and a failure to take the steps required by the law. These failings, combined with a striking lack of compliance with the Mental Capacity Act, make it clear that the very people this legislation was designed to protect remain at risk.*

(p8)

# Intersectionality: health and diversity

Crenshaw's (1989) original use of the term intersectionality was to explain the intersecting effects of race and gender on Black women in legal cases, and that the effects of being both female and Black worked together to cause disadvantage in the American legal system. Here, the focus is not only on being female and Black, but other social categories of marginalised groups who experience health inequalities: the LGBTQIA+ community, people with learning disabilities and mental health issues, disabilities, and religions that have a history of being marginalised in Western Christian society, such as Judaism and Islam. Intersectionality can be used as an analytical tool to understand the wider context of the human experience in society (Collins and Bilge, 2016) and in healthcare (Green et al., 2017). The emergence of COVID-19 has emphasised how the intersecting effects of age, gender, ethnicity and other social categories have been significantly impacted on causing worsening clinical outcomes for patients and healthcare professionals.

## Case study: an Asian woman with learning disabilities

Jatinder Kaur is a 25-year-old British Asian Sikh woman with a mild learning disability who lives at home with her parents. She has a good support network of her parents, family and friends, a full social life, and a part-time job. She is admitted to a surgical ward with moderate to severe lower abdominal pain, nausea, and vomiting. Jatinder's pain is not being controlled effectively; she is crying out periodically in an unusual way, and her family are worried and concerned as they have never seen her behave like this when unwell, and have informed the nurse that this indicates something seriously wrong. Matthew is the registered nurse working in the bay of patients in which Jatinder is located. He is finding it difficult to manage all the relatives calling the ward as no visitors are allowed due to the

COVID-19 lockdown rules at the time. It is hard to interpret her behaviour in relation to pain, especially with intravenous morphine having been given for the pain 30 minutes ago. He has nursed 'Asian patients' before and a few patients who have learning disabilities, and Jatinder is not acting in the way he is expecting.

The intersecting issues here are ethnicity, culture, religion, learning disabilities and gender. Together they can make the 'perfect storm' of discrimination, leading to poor care delivery and outcome for Jatinder's care. Non-white patients and those with learning disabilities have poorer health outcomes (Emerson et al., 2016; Kavanagh et al., 2021) based on institutional racism, racial unconscious bias, prejudice, and discrimination by health professionals and the NHS as an organisation (Drewniak et al., 2017; FitzGerald and Hurst, 2017). Jatinder's ability to convey her needs to healthcare professionals based on her learning disability and family members or carers not being listened to means that the assessment of care around pain management can be poor, which increases her risk of deteriorating without the appropriate interventions. Women's accounts of presenting symptoms, particularly B&B women, have been problematised by the assessment and planning of care not being appropriate for their needs (Andrews et al., 2017).

## Research summary: unconscious bias and racism in healthcare

The goal for healthcare professionals is to consistently deliver safe, competent care equitably to all patients (NMC, 2018a). Individualised patient-centred care delivery is the cornerstone of modern healthcare (Ryan, 2022). Unconscious bias, or implicit bias as it can also be called, is a significant barrier to achieving this (Holm et al., 2017). We all have biases and stereotypes about people and groups that can be based on culture (Schultz and Baker, 2017), race and ethnicity (Holm et al., 2017), and physical and mental impairment. Bucknor-Ferron and Zagaja (2016) define unconscious bias as *the multifaceted evaluation of one group and its members relative to another* (p61). The evaluation is unconscious; you are not directly aware that you are delivering care inadequately because of negative stereotyping based on preconceived ideas and expectations of an individual or group's behaviour.

There is also a train of thought that it is more than unconscious bias and individual actions when it comes to the differences in the experience of healthcare and the disproportionally worse health outcomes for B&B patients. Systemic racism in healthcare is an issue (Essex et al., 2022). When looking at the determinants of health in Chapter 2, a closer look at systemic racism will take place.

For the moment you, as a healthcare professional, must look at yourself and those around you in clinical practice. Care can be poor because of unconscious bias affecting clinical decision-making and interactions between patient and healthcare professional, and within the systems and processes of a health organisation and its staff (FitzGerald and Hurst, 2017; Kapur, 2015).

Activity 1.3 looks at a clinical encounter where unconscious bias could impact negatively on decision-making.

## Activity 1.3   Reflection

Think about how you expect a person to behave in certain circumstances:

- when they are a patient in pain;
- a postpartum mother who tells you that they feel something is wrong with them;
- when they are a grieving relative; and
- when a 75-year-old patient is being taught how to take their blood glucose level.

Now think about how ethnicity, age, sexuality, learning disability, or religion added to any of these situations might change how you behave in each of these cases without you even thinking that they do. If that behaviour discriminates against that patient or family members in a negative way, that behaviour could be attributed to unconscious bias. This in turn can have a negative effect on the patient's experience, healthcare delivery, and health outcome.

*An outline of what you might find is given at the end of the chapter.*

Bucknor-Ferron and Zagaja (2016) ask healthcare professionals to consider the following points in order to reduce unconscious bias:

- *Personal awareness and acknowledgement*: an ability to look at yourself and be aware that you hold these biases.
- *Empathy*: an ability to understand what your patients are feeling and experiencing.
- *Advocacy*: supporting your patients as they move through the health service.
- *Education*: learning formally on your course and learning from others and yourself from your own experiences.

These are attributes that, as a student in nursing or midwifery, you should be fine-tuning, and will continue to do so throughout your career. The COVID-19 pandemic has only highlighted even more why these attributes and abilities are so important.

Let us now look at what you have gained from this chapter.

## Chapter summary

This chapter has considered the concept of diversity, what it means in terms of various social groups within the UK, and how its meaning has changed. The chapter has introduced important terms, such as 'race', 'culture', 'ethnicity', 'unconscious bias', racism, and

BLM. Also considered was how older age may be a factor. The vital importance of the social determinants of health has been discussed, showing how they can lead to poor health outcomes for patients from diverse backgrounds such as LGBTQIA+, and people who are disabled or have a learning disability. Finally, the chapter introduced the term 'intersectionality' as a means of linking together different aspects of people's identities. We saw how, without an understanding of intersectionality, it can increase the risk of poor clinical decision-making and lead to inequity and inequality of care.

# Activities: brief outline answers

## Activity 1.1    Reflection (p12)

Think of how ethnic diversity could affect care delivery.

Racial discrimination, Islamophobia, ageism, and unconscious bias can lead healthcare professionals to make poor clinical decisions due to how you or colleagues may behave towards these groups detrimentally, making poor clinical decisions or restricting access to services.

An example of what you might have witnessed could be the treatment of a young African Caribbean man with mental health problems seen as more threatening and violent than his white male counterpart in an emergency department, a ward, or in the patient's home; the assumption that an older person cannot learn new skills or has some form of cognitive impairment and speaking only to family members and not the older patient; not listening to B&B pregnant women's concerns without sufficient clinical data to make a safe clinical decision and the reasoning being based on gender and ethnicity and how seriously that information may be taken.

It is important to have sufficient knowledge of how some ethnic groups are more susceptible to specific health-related issues (e.g. genetic conditions such as sickle-cell anaemia in people of African and Caribbean descent, or an increased risk of prostate cancer in African Caribbean men – one in four – compared to white men – one in eight, and maternal deaths of B&B women – Asian – two times – Black women – five times – who are more likely to die than white women).

## Activity 1.2    Evidence-based practice and research (p14)

The six statements are as follows:

Statement 1 People from Black, Asian, and other Minority Ethnic groups have their views represented in setting priorities and designing local health and well-being programmes.

Statement 2 People from Black, Asian, and other Minority Ethnic groups are represented in peer and lay roles within local health and well-being programmes.

Statement 3 People from Black, Asian, and other Minority Ethnic groups at high risk of type 2 diabetes are referred to an intensive lifestyle change programme.

Statement 4 People from Black, Asian, and other Minority Ethnic groups referred to a cardiac rehabilitation programme are given a choice of times and settings for the sessions and are followed up if they do not attend.

Statement 5 People from Black, Asian, and other Minority Ethnic groups can access mental health services in a variety of community-based settings.

Statement 6 People from Black, Asian, and other Minority Ethnic groups with a serious mental illness have a physical health assessment at least annually.

If you are working in an area that has a high B&B population, it is in the best interests of your patients that you are familiar with this type of evidence-based information with which to make an appropriate decision, offer health advice and include your patient in their care.

## Activity 1.3    Reflection (p18)

There are differences in how cultural and ethnic groups as well as genders express pain and are assessed for pain. If your expectation is not attuned to this, you may not assess pain levels appropriately, and this could have serious patient care implications.

You might react inappropriately to different expressions of grief by a bereaved person, which can worsen the experience of the death of a loved one.

You might have an expectation that certain ethnic groups or older patients are going to be more 'hard work' or 'difficult to teach' due to their age.

## Further reading

**Bucknor-Ferron, P and Zagaja, L** (2016) Five strategies to combat unconscious bias. *Nursing,* 46(11): 61–2.

This article is an excellent piece on unconscious bias in healthcare. The writers identify groups that unconscious bias affects and the different types of bias that exist, as well as how unconscious bias affects clinical decisions and what as health professionals we can try to do to eliminate it from our decision-making.

**Hassen, N, Lofters, A, Michael, S, Mall, A, Pinto, AD, and Rackal, J** (2021). Implementing anti-racism interventions in healthcare settings: a scoping review. *International Journal of Environmental Research and Public Health*, 18(6), 2993.

This article discusses some important issues on racism and healthcare, what is being done and what could be done to stop this in healthcare using varied anti-racist strategies.

**Scriven, A** (2017) *Ewles & Simnett's Promoting Health: A Practical Guide* (7th edn). Oxford: Elsevier Health.

This is a well-established book in the field of health promotion, and Chapter 2 has some important points to make on the inequalities of health in an accessible and informative way.

## Useful websites

Royal College of Nursing (2020) Fair care for Trans and Non-Binary People

**www.rcn.org.uk/Professional-Development/publications/rcn-fair-care-trans-non-binary-uk-pub-009430**

*Build Back Fairer: The COVID-19 Marmot Review: The Pandemic, Socioeconomic and Health Inequalities in England Fair Society Healthy Lives*

**www.nhsggc.org.uk/media/270160/build-back-fairer-the-covid-19-marmot-review.pdf**

This is an important report that deserves further reading as it gives a COVID-19-related discussion of health inequality in the UK. Professor Sir Michael Marmot is highly respected in the field of inequality and health and has researched and written extensively on inequalities in health.

Mencap:

**www.mencap.org.uk/learning-disability-explained/what-learning-disability**

This is the website for the charity whose main objective is to support people and their families with learning disabilities (LDs). This page looks at some issues discussed in this chapter. It is useful for healthcare professionals and the public alike. It has information on projects run for people with LDs to research and statistics on how to improve the lives and care required for people with LDs.

SCOPE:

**www.scope.org.uk/**

Scope primary function is to gain equality for people with a disability. It is the disability equality charity in England and Wales, providing practical information, statistics, projects, and emotional support when it's most needed, and campaigns to create a fairer and more inclusive society for the disabled.

Office for National Statistics (ONS):

**www.ons.gov.uk/**

The ONS is the UK's largest independent producer of official statistics and the recognised national statistical institute of the UK. It is the organisation that collates the data from the population census that is collected every ten years. For a breakdown of the population by ethnic origin, if born in the UK or outside the UK, age range of the population, gender breakdown, and issues related to health, this is the place to go.

World Health Organization (WHO):

**www.who.int**

The WHO began when its constitution came into force on 7 April 1948, and works with its 194 member states, across six regions, from more than 150 offices. WHO staff are united in a shared commitment to achieving better health for everyone, everywhere. They strive to combat diseases – communicable diseases such as COVID-19, influenza, and HIV, and non-communicable diseases such as cancer and heart disease. For ideas of how UK health concerns relate to international health, this is an invaluable resource.

NHS Race and Health Observatory:

**www.nhsrho.org/**

The NHS Race and Health Observatory works to identify and tackle ethnic inequalities in health and care by facilitating research, making health policy recommendations, and enabling long-term transformational change.

# Chapter 2 · Diversity and cultural concepts of health

### Beverley Brathwaite

## NMC Future Nurse: Standards of Proficiency for Registered Nurses

This chapter will address the following platforms and proficiencies:

**Platform 1: Being an accountable professional**

1.4 demonstrate an understanding of, and the ability to challenge, discriminatory behaviour

1.9 understand the need to base all decisions regarding care and interventions on people's needs and preferences, recognising and addressing any personal and external factors that may unduly influence their decisions.

**Platform 2: Promoting health and preventing ill health**

2.2 demonstrate knowledge of epidemiology, demography, genomics and the wider determinants of health, illness and well-being and apply this to an understanding of global patterns of health and well-being outcomes.

**Platform 7: Coordinating care**

7.9 facilitate equitable access to healthcare for people who are vulnerable or have a disability, demonstrate the ability to advocate on their behalf when required, and make necessary reasonable adjustments to the assessment, planning and delivery of their care.

## Chapter aims

After reading this chapter, you will be able to:

- explain what health is and how it relates to diverse members of the population;
- define the terms 'epidemiology', 'demography', and 'genomics';

- understand how power in relation to racism, prejudice, discrimination, and stereotyping affects healthcare outcomes for diverse groups; and
- understand determinants of health and inequality of health, and the impact of these within diverse groups.

# Introduction

## Case study: Cunningham Street continued

Let us go back to Cunningham Street, with its inhabitants of differing ethnicities, cultures, faiths, religions, sexualities, and intellectual abilities. Anish, of Asian descent, lives at number 35, and his wife is due for her first annual smear test. Karen at number 12, who is white, has been experiencing vaginal discharge for the past month and is worried, but she is reluctant to go to the GP as the practice nurse previously asked questions about her personal life with her wife. A middle-aged man who identifies as Roma is experiencing ongoing joint pain and is trying to get an appointment at the GP practice at the end of the road. At number 2, Olufunke's mother, who is of Nigerian descent, has high blood pressure. At number 5, Jennifer, who is a young woman of Caribbean descent and is on the autistic spectrum, is worried about her friend Jordan, who is of dual heritage and who is struggling to manage her new life following a below-knee amputation.

These residents on Cunningham Street all have health needs that require evidence-based clinical knowledge that is specific to their ethnicity, culture, sexuality, disability, and intellectual abilities.

In this chapter, we will be addressing health as a concept, and how it has changed over time, as well as looking at how the experiences of health and healthcare differ between members of the community. There have been some changes on Cunningham Street since the COVID-19 pandemic arrived in early 2020 and its residents have experienced multiple lockdowns, working from home, and delayed treatments (along with the emotional and psychological impact of this). The impact of the pandemic on 'normal' healthcare delivery, health outcomes, and negative experiences that can occur from within the NHS, as well as the drivers for these experiences, will be examined. We will also consider health both internationally and nationally from a diversity perspective. People from communities such as those that have been discussed already are more susceptible to certain health conditions, outcomes, experiences of healthcare, and differing life expectancy than the general population. Reasons for inequitable outcomes, such as COVID-19, determinants of health, institutional racism, and stereotyping based on ethnicity, gender, LGBTQIA+ people, disability, and LD will also be examined. The legislation used to combat discrimination and the terminology used will be addressed.

# What is health?

Many people in contemporary times regard health as one of the most precious values in life (Nordenfelt, 2007). However, for some diverse groups, health is experienced in different ways. It is important to understand how stigma, determinants of health, and social determinants can influence the health outcomes and personal experiences of culturally diverse patients. It is influenced by national/international evidence and guidance, and individual interactions. It may seem that you have little control over all of this, but you have more influence than you think. As student nurses, you represent the NHS every day and your interaction with patients makes a significant difference. This should never be underestimated. The more positive the interactions are between you and your patients and their families, significant others, or carers, the bigger the effect on their health in the short and long term. Therefore, this chapter will endeavour to bring together international ideas and key terms that heavily influence national legislation, policy, and care delivery that affect all patients and service users. It will take into consideration the distinctive needs of certain diverse groups. First, let us look at the idea of what 'health' means and how this has changed over time by considering definitions from a variety of organisations:

> *A state of complete physical, mental, and social well-being, and not merely the absence of disease and infirmity.*
>
> (WHO, 1948)

> *A healthy person is someone with the opportunity for meaningful work, secure housing, stable relationships, high self-esteem and healthy behaviours. A healthy society, in turn, is not one that waits for people to become ill, but one that sees how health is shaped by social, cultural, political, economic, commercial, and environmental factors, and acts on these for current and future generations.*
>
> (Health Foundation, 2018, p7)

> *A structural, functional, and emotional state that is compatible with effective life as an individual and as a member of society.*
>
> (McCartney et al., 2019, p9)

There has been a shift away from the term 'complete' used by the World Health Organization (WHO, 1948), which would indicate that if you have a manageable long-term condition, you can be considered healthy. Health is not static and will need to incorporate cultural factors and the ability for people to re-establish a sense of well-being that may have shifted due to physical, mental, and social changes (Naidoo and

Willis, 2022). The transformation of what health can mean has coincided with the change in the diversity of the population both internationally and here in the UK. In parts of the country, differing ethnic, cultural, and religious groups interact with each other as never before. The Health Foundation (2018) gives a broader idea of health within the context of the patient being a member of society, focusing on how that person interacts in society, and considers what can be done to reduce ill health before it happens, with a clear acknowledgement of how society can shape how this happens. McCartney et al. (2019) consider society but appreciate that an individual is a member of society and that the two are inexplicably linked. COVID-19 highlighted the issue of the individual and society in relation to following lockdown restrictions or taking the COVID-19 vaccine – both are based on an individual's health choice, but affect the health of not only the individual but the population as a whole.

Demography and health can give us a better understanding of the distribution of health within a given region and group. With this information, decisions about how, where, and on whom resources are spent can be made. We will take some time to look at health issues related to some of these groups.

# Gypsy, Roma, and Travellers

GRTs are now part of the census data; they were finally added as an ethnic group in the 2011 census. The current estimated size of the population is between 100,000 and 500,000 (Parliament UK, 2019). There has been continued research taking place into their healthcare needs, including older members of the community (Burchardt et al., 2018; Lane et al., 2019).

There are multiple issues related to health and social exclusion that are experienced by GRTs. They are more prone to long-term conditions, and have a higher perinatal infant mortality rate of all ethnic minority populations, as well as higher levels of stress, anxiety, depression, and smoking, and increased alcohol consumption (Cromarty, 2018; Gill et al., 2013). They suffer poorer physical health and poorer access to health and primary care services (EHRC, 2016a). For the GRT community, accessing healthcare is difficult. One reason is their nomadic lifestyle, which means that registering with a GP, and even access to a dentist, can be a challenge. The health issues for this community run throughout the life span from birth, with this group having the highest maternal death rate of any ethnic group, and young children are more at risk due to lower immunisation rates. GRTs live in caravans and houses and still experience *accommodation insecurity* which leads to serious poor health outcomes (Sovacool and Del Rio, 2022).

Greenfields (2017, p25) identified practical and administrative challenges for GRTs, as well as a lack of appropriate documentation, including adequate citizenship documentation, which affects entitlement to services following recent migration and entitlement to welfare. Limited access to or awareness of NHS entitlement is exacerbated by low literacy levels. It is also worth adding that evidence has identified fear of racist attacks and abuse, and racial discrimination and prejudice which worsen their interactions with society and healthcare (Taylor and Hinks, 2021; Lane et al., 2019). More on the experiences of GRT can be found in Chapter 7.

# LGBTQIA+

The term LGBTQIA+ covers a wide range of communities that have similar and differing needs and differing levels of understanding of those needs. For example, is the life of a trans woman the same as a gay man's? It's important to remember that although many communities regrettably face disadvantages and discrimination, this does not mean that their needs are the same. As with any patient, asking questions is important, but more important is what and how you ask. What a patient would like to be called is an obvious first encounter question, but we also need to think about what pronouns our patients want to be identified as and when told follow this through consistently.

Globally, the LGBTQIA+ community must combat discrimination, violence, and criminalisation as same-sex relationships are illegal in 69 UN member states (ILGA, 2020b). Although transgender people have existed across history and cultures throughout the world, transgenderism and transsexualism are considered abnormal in many societies as they diverge from the predominant normative male–female binary that exists across the world (Wylie et al., 2016). The United Nations High Commissioner for Human Rights states that human rights law is obligated to protect all people from discrimination on the grounds of gender identity. This is not always the case, and to determine the experiences of the LGBTQIA+ community in the UK, the Government Equalities Office carried out a national survey in 2018 (see link in useful websites for results of the survey). Possibly based on this information and the British Mental Health Association clearly being against all types of conversion therapy, the British Government are looking into the legalities of conversion therapy.

In relation to Platform 7.13 of the NMC Code, it is necessary for you, as a student, to appreciate the political context and wider determinants of health from which your patients come and in which they find themselves with you and the NHS. For example, the fear of physical violence is an unacceptable reality for many in the LGBTQIA+ community in Europe and the UK (Clark, 2014). The damaging effects of hate crimes against members of the LGBTQIA+ community not only affect their physical but also their emotional and psychological well-being (Jurcic, 2016). Your first encounter with an LGBTQIA+ patient could be in the emergency department, where physical needs would need to be addressed, but where it could also be an opportunity to help with emotional and psychological needs. When a trans person is going for reassignment surgery a non-judgemental and open approach will only benefit their journey. Overall, heterosexuals fare better in healthcare, while bisexuals have the worst experiences, and gay and lesbian people have poorer mental health (Booker et al., 2017). In the longer term, it may be that mental health services are best suited to support the emotional and psychological trauma that can result from experiences of being part of the LGBTQIA+ community. For example, there is a higher risk of suicide and attempted suicide (Peate, 2016). This must not be underestimated as a significant and possible outcome if appropriate support and interventions are not put in place. Bachmann and Gooch (2019), the RCN (2016), and Robinson (2019) have acknowledged the discrimination that LGBTQIA+ patients experience from healthcare professionals. The RCN (2016) has provided a clear policy to reduce this discrimination. It is your responsibility and accountability once registered with the NMC to deliver care equitably. Bristowe et al. (2018) found that the impact of discrimination on the LGBTQIA+ community's health covers their life span. They have a higher risk of some cancers and greater all-cause mortality than heterosexual people. They often present later in the treatment and disease pathway, have unmet bereavement needs, and have a higher rate of mental illness and risky behaviours (e.g. drinking, smoking, drug use) that are linked to discrimination. This discrimination could lead to a reluctance to seek and adhere to effective follow-up or community care and to experiencing poor levels of care while in treatment (Glasper, 2016; RCN, 2016). During COVID-19, self-harming increased due to the social isolation caused by lockdown measures (Phillips, 2021). The effects caused by lockdown and continued discrimination will require you as a nurse to create welcoming and non-judgemental encounters and environments for these service users.

# Learning disabilities

A learning disability (LD) is a reduced intellectual ability and an increased difficulty with everyday activities – for example, household tasks, socialising, or managing money – which affects someone for their whole life.

People with a learning disability tend to take longer to learn and may need support to develop new skills, understand complicated information, and interact with other people (Mencap, 2022). The term intellectual disability is also used (Cluley, 2018).

Current research has found that health and social care professionals do not feel comfortable working with people with learning disabilities due to a lack of knowledge about their needs (Ee et al., 2021). Feeling uncomfortable and having diminished knowledge will absolutely impact on the problem-solving and decision-making of clinical teams and their care delivery to patients with LDs. Evidence also indicates that the reasons for the poorer health of people with intellectual disabilities primarily fall within two broad spheres. First, a range of secondary health conditions is associated with the specific causes of intellectual disabilities. Second, people with intellectual disabilities are much more likely than their non-disabled peers to be exposed to a range of well-established social determinants of poorer health (e.g. poverty, social exclusion, discrimination, and reduced access to timely and effective healthcare) and a lower life expectancy (LE) than those without a LD (University of Bristol, 2021). These are the stark and unacceptable realities of children and adults with LDs. British adults with a LD have a distinctly poorer quality of health than their non-disabled peers (Scottish Learning Disabilities Observatory, 2021). There is also a higher relationship between physical and mental health problems among those with LDs than among the general population (Hatton et al., 2017). As a student nurse of any field, adult, child, mental health, and of course LD, it is extremely likely that you will be providing care for a patient with a LD, and in a variety of different sites of care delivery poor patient safety outcomes continue to be an issue and it is for us as nurses to do better (Louch et al., 2021). A therapeutic relationship between patients who have a LD and their caregiver/support system is an important aspect of care that is crucial for creating and maintaining a safe environment. The community setting is also an area for care delivery for many patients with a LD in their homes and specialised care facilities. The multidisciplinary team (MDT) is, not surprisingly, frequently utilised in care delivery with patients who have mild to severe LDs.

As a member of the MDT, it is important that you know the other members and their role in delivering care holistically to the patient, carers, and family. You will need to know when to refer and the reason for the referral. Activity 2.1 will allow you to think about which members of the MDT are involved.

## Activity 2.1   Teamworking

Make a list of the MDT members who can be involved in the care of patients with learning disabilities and what role they would take in their care.

*An outline of what you might find is given at the end of the chapter.*

Activity 2.1 demonstrates that you must have identified multiple members of the MDT with whom you have worked already or know of the vital role they play. The need to work as a member of the healthcare team in providing the best possible care for this group of patients is an ongoing skill, as new roles are developed particularly to enhance care for patients with learning disabilities.

Due to medical and societal advancement, there has been an increase in the life expectancy of people with LDs (Welsh Government, 2018; Dolan et al., 2021). However, members of the population with LDs continue to have a lower life expectancy than the general population (Dolan, 2021). The mortality rate of people with LDs is complex and incorporates issues of age, gender, ethnicity, deprivation, and type of LD. Table 2.1 highlights some of the common causes of mortality and the relationship between health problems associated with having a LD.

| Health Problem | Cause of Death |
|---|---|
| Neurological disorders – Epilepsy | Seizures / convulsion |
| Dementia | |
| Gastrointestinal problems | Aspiration |
| | Constipation |
| | Colorectal cancer |
| Respiratory problems | Bacterial and aspiration pneumonia |
| | COVID-19 |
| | Lung Cancer |
| Cardiac circulatory problems | Congenital cardiac dysfunction |

*Table 2.1*   Health problems and cause of death associated with learning disability (Tyrer et al., 2022; University of Bristol, 2021)

Due to these complex issues, many people with LDs can have more obstacles to identifying health problems and getting treatment for them. For example, autism can be identified as a LD (although some argue it is not) but understanding an individual's detailed, long-term diagnosis, where they are on the autistic spectrum and how this impacts them both physically and mentally is essential for giving individual patient care (O'Brien and Pearson, 2004).

Annual LD health checks have been a key part of NHS plans to improve care and health for people with LDs and reduce premature mortality since 2008, but unfortunately some evidence suggests it has not helped to reduce the mortality rate (Tryer et al., 2022). Communication, as well as patients not understanding what is happening to them and why, can make it difficult for you to make an accurate clinical decision. There are many identifiable types of LD, for example, Down's Syndrome, but there is not always a physical attribute that may indicate that a LD affects your patient. Even if there is such an attribute, it can be challenging to ascertain the individual's level of understanding of what they are being told or asked. This could easily be misunderstood as incomprehension or uncooperativeness. Hatton et al. (2017) state that *there may be uncertainty over patients' capacity to consent to interventions and a lack of understanding of the legal requirements for proxy decision-making if they cannot* (p24). This is another area where the family, caregivers, and support workers are vital to aid this process. Areas of best practice in which to aid care delivery to patients with LDs have been identified as:

- *Taking a person-centred approach to care and support.*
- *'Joined-up' working with good communication between those involved.*
- *The involvement of families.*
- *Responsiveness to a change in a person's health.*

(University of Bristol, 2020).

## Activity 2.2  Evidence-based practice and research

What is a learning disability? We have discussed a lot about people with LDs but what exactly are LDs and is there any other terminology that can be used instead of or with LDs?

Find the answers to the following questions on the NHS and Gov.uk websites:

1.  What is a learning disability?
2.  What causes LDs?
3.  What does PMLD stand for?

Having gone through this process you will see how multifaceted both the LD community and the terminology used to describe it is.

*An outline of the answers is given at the end of the chapter.*

There is an unfortunate similarity in the health outcomes and experiences of patients with LDs and other forms of disability, as we will look at now.

# Disability

As with other communities, the term 'disability' covers a wide range of characteristics. Historically disability was thought of as a direct consequence of sin or fault or arising due to some inadequacy of the individual (Bunbury, 2019). As they should, contemporary ideas around disabilities have changed but these old ideas still linger and influence how people with disabilities are treated today. The Equality Act defines disability as a physical or mental impairment, where the impairment has a substantial and long-term adverse effect on the ability to carry out normal day-to-day activities (Equality Act, 2010). Consider what we as healthcare professionals think about this definition, or what the patient/service user thinks. Our ideas could be very different, and you must remember that patients may see themselves differently from you as they have every right to. It is the healthcare professional's duty both professionally, legally, and as a member of society to see beyond the disability and see the whole person. There are also hidden disabilities that are not physically apparent. One example would be someone going through cancer treatment. Smith (2021, p74) gives a useful discussion on her personal journey with cancer and how she was treated by friends and colleagues. One of the main areas for her and others is 'that many disabilities are misunderstood and the lack of understanding and awareness results in discrimination'.

The following scenario gives an example of an adolescent with a new disability and how you would try and address not only the physical but the emotional needs.

## Scenario: Jordan, a teenager newly disabled

Jordan Owusu, who is 16, had a below-knee amputation at the beginning of the first COVID-19 lockdown due to osteosarcoma in the lower tibia bone. They are finding rehab and managing their new life difficult both emotionally and physically. Unfortunately, the amputation wound has broken down due to infection. You are a children and young people's student nurse in your second year and have gone with your practice assessor (PA) to review the wound on the ward. Jordan had to be admitted for intravenous antibiotics and monitoring as there was a concern that sepsis could be an issue. When you go to tell Jordan that you would like to renew the dressing, it is obvious that they have recently been crying. You draw the curtains around Jordan, quietly state that it looks like they have been crying and do they want to share why to see if you can help. Jordan says that they are experiencing sadness, anger, and frustration about the amputation, and are worried about how non-disabled people view them, particularly family and friends.

The following activity will help you think about what you can do in more detail.

## Activity 2.3   Decision-making

What do you and your PA do to help, and who else could be involved?

1.   Immediately
2.   Longer term

*An outline of what could be done is given at the end of the chapter.*

The scenario also shows that disability is part of being human. Almost everyone will temporarily or permanently experience disability at some point in their life. Over 1 billion people currently experience disability, with this number increasing due in part to population ageing and an increase in the frequency of non-communicable diseases (WHO, 2022c).

# Diversity: epidemiology, demography, and genomics

There are key terms within Platform 2.2 that deserve to be addressed as they can be aligned with the understanding of issues relating to the changing British population. Demography is the way in which a population is studied to determine the causes of health and disease. Key components of studying the demography of a population are morbidity, mortality, migration, ethnicity, class, and gender. Epidemiology has a close relationship to demography as it is the study of a population and how often disease occurs in different groups within that population (Gurdasani et al., 2019). An example would be to consider a single group – say transgender, women or men, people with LDs or another disability – and then look even closer by separating women by ethnic group or age and determining what disease or illness rates occur in these particular groups, and what targeted prevention or care delivery needs to be arranged. Women over 50 years old should go for breast screening every three years as the risk of breast cancer increases (NHS, 2019). Some Black and Brown (B&B) women are less likely to take up this screening compared to their white counterparts, indicating a need to target campaigns at specific ethnic groups (Baird et al., 2021). Transgender individuals are more at risk of psychological distress and risk of suicide due to stigma-related stress (Bränström and Pachankis, 2020). This is an example of the importance of demographic and epidemiological knowledge in targeting healthcare delivery for diverse groups.

Genomics incorporates and identifies that multiple genes work together with environmental influences, resulting in a situation of health or illness. For example, there is a connection between genetics and pain associated with sickle-cell crisis (Lakkakula et al., 2018). In the case of sickle-cell crisis pain management, nurses will need to appreciate this when assessing a patient for pain.

However, even here there is inequality, as only 2 per cent of the Human Genome Project has been collected from Africa, meaning fewer opportunities to use genomics to aid specific and effective treatments for Africans and patients of African descent (Mabuka-Maroa, 2019).

The pandemic required significant utilisation of epidemiology, demography, and genomics, internationally, for example, by the WHO and nationally by the ONS. Both are used consistently to inform practice and resources such as COVID-19 vaccine testing and access.

In 2020, Genomics England announced that they would begin a study of 20,000 hospitalised patients who had experienced the worst symptoms of COVID-19 and compare them to 15,000 patients who had only mild symptoms. This is an effort to explore potential genomic differences in susceptibility to the disease. The study will take some time to complete, and it is not known how the research will either collect or address other risk factors alongside genetic variability. Similarly, the Biobank longitudinal study in the UK has requested that its current participants enrol in a subsidiary study to examine those factors (genetic or otherwise) that could influence susceptibility to COVID-19, although the proportion of B&B individuals participating in the Biobank study is lower than white people (Bently, 2020).

There are some genetic conditions that in the UK are more likely to be found in B&B people. The activity below encourages you to discover what they are and how they can be treated.

## Activity 2.4   Evidence-based practice and research

Go to the Genomics Education Programme web page on the Health Education England website: www.genomicseducation.hee.nhs.uk/resources/genetic-conditions-factsheets/

Look for the following genetic conditions: sickle-cell anaemia and alpha thalassemia.

Find out:

1.   What ethnic groups are more likely to have the condition?
2.   What is given as the reason for the genetic condition?
3.   What is the clinical management of the condition?

*An outline of what you might find is given at the end of the chapter.*

Some genetic-based conditions have a strong connection to ethnic and cultural groups. Activity 2.4 will get you to look at sickle-cell anaemia and find out more about this genetic condition and the ethnic groups in which it is more likely to be found.

As you can see from Activity 2.4, Health Education England is a resource not only for healthcare professionals, but patients and family members, and it can be used as an additional source of information. Accessing varied forms of health information in differing formats improves health literacy, particularly for diverse groups. This is looked at in more detail in Chapter 7.

The ethnic demography of an area will increase the possibility of certain genetic conditions being prevalent, and in turn the need for the use of local primary and secondary services. As a nurse working in certain parts of the country, it is in your and your patient's best interests that you are familiar with these genetic conditions to ensure that competent care can be given. These are conditions that will require lifelong support and medical and nursing interventions not only for the physical symptoms, but the psychological symptoms that can coexist with them, such as depression (Jonassaint et al., 2016). There is also a cultural context. For example, patients with sickle-cell anaemia can have negative experiences in hospital services and care delivery (Haywood et al., 2014). These patients and their family members can feel shame, blame themselves, or see sickle-cell anaemia as a curse (Buser et al., 2021). As a nurse, it is your responsibility to respond to these ideas in a respectful manner and to support patients in moving away from these negative feelings. Giving clear information on the genetic reasons for sickle-cell anaemia, as well as referring to the appropriate specialist nurse in the hospital and within the community to ensure continued support, is of paramount importance to the ongoing well-being of patients with sickle-cell anaemia.

It is necessary to recognise that a genetic link is specifically based on a mutated missing or additional gene causing a diagnosable health problem. 'Race' and ethnicity are not completely linked to genetics – 'race' is socially constructed and largely signifies a complex mixture of behavioural, environmental, and social exposures (Seewoodhary, 2021). Although diabetes, hypertension, and prostate cancer are more prevalent in B&B ethnic communities, we must be careful not to engage in biological racism (the idea that there is an innate biological basis for these medical conditions in B&B people that does not clearly exist). Biological racism omits serious consideration of complex social factors such as poverty, austerity, and varied forms of prejudice that impact on why B&B people are more at risk of certain conditions, including a greater risk of death from COVID-19 (Saini, 2020). It puts the focus on health completely on the individual and does not address the associated social, socio-economic, and political causes of poor health.

This is a good place to look closely at the social reasons for poor health, particularly forms of prejudice and stigmatisation.

# Stigma

Let us take a moment to discuss stigmatisation. Stigma refers to the negative regard, inferior status, and relative powerlessness that society collectively accords to people who possess a particular characteristic or who belong to a particular group or category (Frost, 2011). If we reflect back on the social groups we have looked at already, stigma can definitely be a contributing factor to how they sadly continue to be treated and their lived experiences of disadvantage and discrimination in society and healthcare.

In this chapter, we have looked at the LGBTQIA+, GRT, LD, disability, and B&B communities. In one way or another, all of the groups we have looked at experience stigma, discrimination, stereotyping, or other significant social constructs, such as racism. The LGBTQIA+ community faces so much stigmatisation that they fear informing health professionals of their sexuality because they have experienced homophobia (Rostosky et al., 2021). In turn, this fear means people are more likely to approach a health professional later in the progress of symptoms and illness (Richman and Hatzenbuehler, 2014). In the LD community, stigma not only harms care for the patient, but the family can also be stigmatised. Werner and Shulman (2015) call this *stigma by association* (p272). As a result, the voiced concerns of the family and main carers of people with a LD may be ignored, with disastrous consequences, which has led to the unnecessary deaths of patients with LDs (University of Bristol, 2021). The GRT community experiences racism, discrimination, and being stigmatised at an unprecedented level. They experience social deprivation, low literacy, and educational attainment (Sovacool and Del Rio, 2022). The NHS and healthcare professionals encounter significant challenges to meet the complex GRT healthcare needs caused by these experiences. Healthcare professionals can be judgemental, and their lack of cultural awareness is likely to be influenced by the media reinforcing stereotypes of poor behaviour and bad attributes of the GRT community (EHRC, 2016a). As with other minority groups, this can lead to them accessing health services later in the progression of their health problem, and consequently poorer outcomes from treatment.

You must take into consideration prejudice when defining racism. *Prejudice is the property of all people, but racism can be attributed only to those who have the power to translate their prejudices into action* (Baxter, 1988, p3). The health service as an organisation has the power to implement practices that offer equality but are not equitable. In the following section, we will look at how forms of racism impact healthcare.

# Racisms and bias in healthcare

Before addressing racisms, some understanding of what constitutes 'race' is required. 'Race' is a social construct and there is no biological basis to it. This must be acknowledged and understood as a concept if there is to be any attempt to seriously address the real issue of racisms in healthcare (Hamed et al., 2020). Stating 'racisms' and not racism here is to acknowledge that there are different forms of racisms and biases. The addition of BLM to academic discussions on racism in health is an indication of how global racism is, which it has always been, and frames it in a way that positions the B&B experience as central. This is not to the detriment or exclusion of any other group, but an examination of the evidence in healthcare consistently indicates that B&B groups face health inequalities due to racism (Essex et al., 2020).

Baxter (1988) states the following on institutional racism within the NHS:

> *Institutional racism means racism is embedded in organisational structures. There are various ways in which racism is maintained and reinforced within British institutions. Firstly, there is racism which operates through default. Here the institution adheres to the traditional way of doing things, ignoring the multiracial and multicultural nature of the society it is now called upon to serve. Secondly, within the institution there are people in positions of power who are not consciously racist, but who are nevertheless influenced by racist stereotypes. Thirdly, racism occurs in institutions through the rules and regulations which, although they appear neutral, have the effect to exclude Black people while maintaining the privileged position of whites.*

> (Baxter, 1988, p4–5)

> *Racism acts as a barrier to the creation of better healthcare systems.*

> (Russell, 2022, p11)

These two quotes are over 30 years apart but unfortunately the underlying problem of racism and its impact on the NHS and health continues. This more recent idea about how racism impacts health continues to appreciate that systems within institutions are a factor, not only individual action. However, we are all part of institutions and either formulate or follow systems. Whether racism is systemic or individual in healthcare, one does not function without the other.

The existence of racism in healthcare is about individual practitioners making racially based decisions, unconsciously or consciously, through bias. If the outcome means poor treatment, healthcare cannot be fully effective for all who use it. This leads to social and health disadvantages causing the social determinant of health to have a racial component (Marmot et al., 2020a).

As a student, you may already have witnessed this in the clinical setting in the varied interactions that take place between the nurse, patient, and significant others such as family carers and support workers. Without a clear understanding of how stigma, unconscious or conscious bias, or racial stereotypes work, a patient's treatment, or any attempt at altering the way diverse individuals and groups are treated in the NHS, will never change, and unacceptable clinical decisions will continue to be made. You must look at your own conscious and unconscious biases and racist stereotyping of your patients. This is an unacceptable practice that must be worked on constantly as you have a duty of care to your patients that is non-discriminatory. Biases, particularly racial infused, should have no place in your clinical decision-making process and care delivery.

An example of a situation that can arise in the clinical environment can help to give you an idea of how stereotyping and racism, both conscious and unconscious, can influence communication and clinical decisions.

## Scenario: communication

You are a third-year adult nursing student on your final placement before finishing your degree. Olufemi is a 25-year-old Black British man of African descent; he is over six feet tall and well-built, and it looks like he works out regularly. He is admitted overnight to your acute medical ward placement in a sickle-cell crisis. He has not had a severe crisis that required admission to hospital since his teens, and this is his first time being admitted to an adult ward. On the morning shift with your practice supervisor (PS) at handover at 7.30 a.m., he is said to be in a little pain and is 'a bit needy like a lot of "sicklers" are'. He has intravenous morphine prescribed every two hours, which is just about managing his pain, and he has intravenous fluids running over eight hours. When you both go on to the ward after the handover, Olufemi is in terrible pain, particularly in his legs, which have suddenly worsened. He is ringing the bell and calling out in pain when you enter the bay. Your PS goes straight to the call bell and turns it off and tells him to try to be a little quieter as the noise he is making is disturbing the other patients. Before you and your PS have a chance to do anything else, Olufemi angrily states that you are more concerned about the noise he is making than the excruciating pain he is experiencing; he wants some painkillers now, and after this he wants to go home as he would be better off there than in here, where his illness is not understood and 'the care is rubbish'. Your PS replies to the patient that she is going to get the doctor to speak to him and does not engage in any other form of communication with Olufemi. She asks you to take his vital signs and walks away, saying to you, 'I don't have to take being spoken to like that by that type of patient'. You introduce yourself to him and ask if you can take his vital signs; he continues to be angry and says, 'Go the hell away and just get me my painkillers, I can't take this pain anymore'.

From this scenario, we now proceed to Activity 2.5, where you will consider the possible reasons for what happened and why.

## Activity 2.5   Decision-making

From what was said in the handover and by your PS considering issues of gender, ethnicity, and Olufemi's sickle-cell disorder, what is being stigmatised?

- Olufemi is obviously angry. Why do you think this is?
- What could you and your practice supervisor do to improve this situation?

*An outline of what you might answer is given at the end of the chapter.*

In the above scenario and in Activity 2.5, we have looked at the possible experience of a Black man of African descent in the NHS. There sadly has been a real case in which Evan Smith, a young Black man with sickle cell, died due to delayed treatment. The coroner for the case stated: *The delay in treating Mr Smith with a timely exchange transfusion was the cause of his death.* He also went on to say, *although staff provided basic medical care, it was the 'wrong' care* (BBC, 2021).

There may never be a clear reason for what impacted the decision-making of the healthcare professionals looking after Evan Smith, but the sad loss of this young man's life illustrates the importance of not letting stigma or stereotyping influence your willingness to listen to a patient. Being prepared to develop an understanding of the individual experience of a condition is vital and reflection may help you to understand the impact of not doing so.

# Social determinants of health in the UK

Many different factors contribute to a person's current state of health. Marmot et al.'s (2020a) report lists some of the areas considered as social determinants of health, and some of the main points are highlighted below in Figure 2.1.

| Children in their early years and young people – poverty, childcare workforce, schooling, free school meals, youth crime, school exclusion, funding for schools |
|---|
| Work and employment – pay, quality of work and in-work poverty |
| Food and fuel insecurity and poverty |
| Austerity – funding cuts |
| Housing |
| Transport |
| Climate change |

*Figure 2.1*　Some social determinants of health

Our patients come from parts of our local areas that experience these social determinants of health to varying degrees. Physical social environments and deprivation differ greatly, therefore having an idea about the population that your clinical environment serves will give you a sense of why they are unwell and what can be done to support them in the short and long term, particularly if they have a long-term condition. Life expectancy (LE) varies greatly across the UK, even within a city, and is an indication of how effective healthcare is and the impact of social determinants of health (Marmot et al., 2021). The LE of the population has not significantly improved in recent years but there is a mixed picture based on gender and ethnicity in the general population (ONS, 2021a).

The World Health Organization (WHO, 2008b) has made it its core business to address social determinants of health internationally. As can be observed, the social determinants of health are only one area covered by the determinants of health. The importance of these social determinants on diverse groups cannot be underestimated.

To give your local area of work some global context, it would be worthwhile looking at the Commission on Social Determinants of Health's final report: *Closing the Gap in a Generation: Health Equity through Action on the Social Determinants of Health* (WHO, 2008b).

In Activity 2.6 we will look at what the WHO has to say about the determinants of health in more detail.

## Activity 2.6　Evidence-based practice and research

Using the link below,
www.who.int/news-room/questions-and-answers/item/determinants-of-health
find the following:

Three determinants of health that the WHO identify as important.

The other seven factors that they consider make people healthy or not.

*An outline of what you should find is given at the end of the chapter.*

Following on from Activity 2.6, social and health determinants are external societal forces that have a huge influence on how well a person succeeds throughout their life span, including ill health. There is only so much the NHS (which is free healthcare at the point of access) can do if inequality in society continues. This does not mean that we, as nurses, should not do our utmost to ensure that care is delivered to a high and equitable standard. We also need to understand how social determinants affect health and that we can signpost patients for support in social care and from the multidisciplinary team.

Going back to the Marmot Reports (Marmot et al., 2020a; Marmot et al., 2020b), they argue that the most effective way to reduce health inequalities is to make changes to the background causes of ill health. There are a lot of complexities in addressing social and health inequalities and Marmot argues that over the last ten years things have actually worsened, with COVID-19 only exacerbating health inequalities (Marmot et al., 2020b; Marmot et al., 2021). We have highlighted that members of society from diverse and marginalised groups add an additional layer to these complexities. Governments, and to a certain extent healthcare, focus on lifestyle interventions or *lifestyle drift* (Marmot et al., 2010, p86). Diverse populations can belong to lower socio-economic groups, which perpetuates the inequalities they face. How much you earn determines where you live, and the education you attain will improve your earnings and your ability to navigate the health and social care systems to benefit your health.

As a healthcare professional, it can appear that our role will have insufficient impact on the health outcomes for diverse groups, but this is not the case. A large, knowledgeable, multidisciplinary workforce is paramount for acting on the social determinants of health. The Marmot Review clearly understands that a shortage of trained healthcare staff to deliver basic functions of service delivery, and to deliver interventions to reduce inequality and improve health outcomes, will cause a *major impediment to success* (Marmot et al., 2010, p88). Therefore, your role as a student nurse is important.

## Social determinants of health and the COVID-19 pandemic

The diagram below illustrates how some groups within the population have been disproportionately affected by COVID-19. As you can see, many of the groups and areas that we've discussed so far are in Figure 2.2. For example, older adults, B&B men, pregnant B&B women, B&B healthcare workers, and people with LDs.

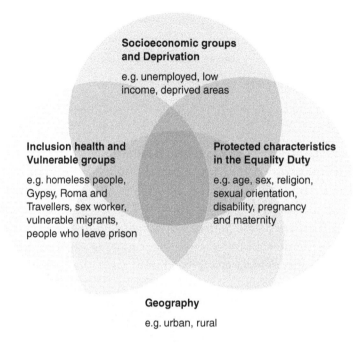

*Figure 2.2*   From Public Health England (2021), *Health Equity Assessment Tool (HEAT): Executive Summary*

There is so much data and evidence on the inequality that exists with social determinants of health and the reasons for certain groups of people having a higher infection and mortality rate due to the COVID-19 pandemic (much of which has been cited in this book). Bentley (2020) takes a detailed look at the structural racism in British society that increased the risk of exposure to COVID-19 for B&B people, such as being a healthcare professional or other essential worker unable to work from home, poor fitting personal protection equipment, and being in urban areas with limited space for social distancing. Phillips (2021) suggests that the available data on LGBTQIA+ risk is due to 'physical health inequity' (p1), such as a potential increase in long-term conditions of the respiratory system and cardiovascular disease due to a higher usage of alcohol and smoking than the general population, and lesbian and bisexual women being more likely to be obese, all which increase the risk of severity of symptoms with COVID-19. Kavanagh et al. (2021, 2022) consider children and adults with LDs and the health and social care systems that were unable to respond effectively to the rapidly evolving needs created by the pandemic. On an individual level, many in the LD community require assistance with personal hygiene and constant supervision, meaning that social distancing was impossible and increased the risk of COVID-19 due to exposure.

# Equality legislation

The Equality Act 2010 collated legislation that already existed covering a variety of areas and older legislation focusing on anti-discriminatory practices in work and society. Ultimately, it identified nine protected characteristics that are unlawful to discriminate against. They are age, disability, gender reassignment, race, religion or belief, sex, sexual orientation, marriage and civil partnership, and pregnancy and maternity. There is a legal framework that acknowledges discrimination exists even within a country that is so diverse.

It is important that, as healthcare professionals, we are aware that there can be legal consequences for organisations, as well as poor health outcomes for patients, if discrimination exists. The Equality Act 2010 is a good place to start looking at the different types of discrimination:

- *Direct discrimination:* This occurs when a person treats another less favourably than they treat, or would treat, others because of a protected characteristic.
- *Indirect discrimination:* This occurs when an apparently neutral policy (provision, criterion or practice) is applied *that puts, or would put, people sharing a protected characteristic at a particular disadvantage, and puts the individual at that disadvantage* (HM Government, 2013).

Reasonable adjustment is part of the Equality Act 2010, and it is Platform 7.9 (NMC, 2018a) which identifies that, as nurses, we must consider what is important and can be changed in order to ensure that when dealing with vulnerable and disabled patients, an appropriate level of care is given. An example of this in practice is that some patients require a nurse to deliver care on a one-to-one basis for the duration of their stay in hospital, or a relative can stay for long periods to be with their family member and provide essential aspects of care independently or with the assistance of a healthcare professional.

## Research summary: gender and age

It is necessary to take a moment to think about issues of gender and age. In health, the biological difference of sex means that women are more likely to have breast cancer than men, but men also get breast cancer (Cancer Research UK, 2020). Trans women and men, depending on whether they have had any bottom or top surgery, are still at risk of sex-specific cancers of the prostate or cervix/womb. These matters would need to be addressed in a respectful and dignified way. In the Equality Act 2010, sex, gender reassignment, sexual orientation and pregnancy are considered protected characteristics (PC). Evidence repeatedly shows that B&B women are more likely to die from complications of pregnancy and childbirth than their white counterparts (MBRRACE-UK, 2021; Birthrights, 2022).

## Chapter summary

This chapter started by discussing the changing emphasis on what is considered health. It then explored crucial healthcare issues related to LD, disability, GRT, and LGBTQIA+ communities, as well as life expectancy differences between diverse communities. The chapter introduced concepts and ideas that you may not have considered in this way before around how they impact patients' experiences of healthcare and having their needs met. The importance of epidemiology and demographic genomics, as well as their effect on diverse groups, was discussed, and we built on Chapter 1's discussion on the relationship between the social determinants of health and health inequalities caused by racisms, conscious and unconscious bias, stigmatisation, prejudice, and discrimination. We looked at the impact of the COVID-19 pandemic on the health of diverse groups and ages. Finally, the legal framework against discrimination that exists in society and healthcare was addressed by looking at the Equality Act 2010.

## Activities: brief outline answers

### Activity 2.1   Teamworking (p28)

It is important to acknowledge the value of a positive and constructive relationship between patients, families, carers, and healthcare professionals. Below is a list (not complete) of the MDT members that could be involved.

- *Consultant (doctor):* LDs cover a broad spectrum of conditions; therefore, the right senior doctor is very important. Specialist knowledge, correct diagnosis, and ongoing care are their role.
- *General practitioner:* Also important to the ongoing care of the patient with an LD in the community.
- *Teacher:* Education and assuring the right type of educational support for a person with an LD needs to be carefully considered due to the varied abilities that a person with an LD may have.
- *Learning disability liaison nurse:* can help with facilitating admissions to hospital for a person with an LD, especially when it is a planned admission (RCN, 2017, p10).
- *Community learning disability teams (CLDTs):* an invaluable resource. They typically comprise of learning disability nurses, psychologists, psychiatrists, speech and language therapists, physiotherapists, occupational therapists, and arts therapists. They normally have an open referral system and are experts in helping people with learning disabilities access various community facilities, especially healthcare (RCN, 2017).

### Activity 2.2   Evidence-based practice and research (p30)

1.   *What is a learning disability?*

A LD, not to be confused with a learning difficulty such as dyslexia or dyspraxia, is a label given to a group of conditions that are present before the age of 18. This impacts on the way individuals develop in all core areas, and ultimately how they live their lives and access healthcare.

A LD needs to be viewed as a *complex way of being* (Gates, 2001).

For simplicity, this document has grouped causes and conditions. The causes of a learning disability mainly fall into three distinct areas:

prenatal period

perinatal period

postnatal period

2.   *What causes learning disabilities?*

We do not always know why a person has a LD. Sometimes it is because a person's brain development is affected, either before they are born, during their birth, or in early childhood. This can be caused by things such as: the mother becoming ill in pregnancy; problems during the birth that stop enough oxygen from getting to the brain; or the unborn baby having some genes passed on from its parents that make having a LD more likely. Other causes include illness, such as meningitis, or injury in early childhood.

There are some health conditions where you may be more likely to have a LD. For example, everyone with Down's Syndrome has some level of LD, and so do many people with cerebral palsy. Some people with epilepsy also have a LD and so do many autistic people.

3.   *What does PMLD stand for?*

A profound and multiple learning disability (PMLD) is when a person has a severe learning disability and other disabilities that significantly affect their ability to communicate and be independent.

Someone with a profound and multiple learning disability might have difficulties seeing, hearing, speaking, and moving. They may have complicated health and social care needs due to these or other conditions.

# Activity 2.3   Decision-making (p31)

What do you and your PA do to help, and who else could be involved?

1.   *Immediately:* Acknowledge their feelings; ask if anything specifically happened today or recently to make them feel this way today; have they been able to express their feelings to family and friends; reassure them feelings are normal; ask if you can tell their parents about how they are feeling; speak to their doctors; refer onto counselling, support groups, websites that might be helpful.

2.   *Longer term involves support groups:* Assure GP is aware of Jordan's feelings on discharge; consider the use of medication in consultation with the psychiatric team; keep reinforcing to the family how important they are as part of their recovery by listening and that Jordan expressing their feelings are helpful and contributes to their recovery both physically and mentally. See if support groups or online groups have been used, and if so, were they helpful?

# Activity 2.4   Evidence-based practice and research (p33)

## Sickle-cell anaemia

*   *What ethnic groups are more likely to have the condition?* Sickle-cell disease is common in people of African, Mediterranean, Middle Eastern, and Indian ancestry, and in people from the Caribbean and parts of Central and South America.

- *What is given as the reason for the genetic condition?* Being a carrier for sickle-cell disease is thought to convey some protection against malaria, and as such there is an increased prevalence of people with sickle-cell traits where malaria is common.
- *What is the clinical management of the condition?* Management guidelines recommend that all patients should receive an optimal level of care delivered close to home, as well as access to clinical experts in specialist centres. In addition, services should support 'expert' patients, parents, and carers in managing the condition at home when appropriate. Multidisciplinary management should aim to prevent and treat infections, pain, and complications, and include social and psycho-educational support. The mainstay of primary prevention is to avoid dehydration, extremes of temperature, physical exhaustion, and extremely high altitude.

## Alpha thalassemia

- *What ethnic groups are more likely to have the condition?* Alpha thalassaemia is most prevalent in sub-Saharan Africa, South and Southeast Asia, the Middle East, and regions of the Mediterranean, such as Cyprus.
- *What is given as the reason for the genetic condition?* The genetic basis of alpha thalassaemia is complex, as each person inherits two alpha-globin genes from each parent. Because of the complexity, referral to specialist clinical genetics services is recommended.
- *What is the clinical management of the condition?* Most patients with HbH disease (alpha thalassaemia) are well but will have a haematological evaluation every 6 to 12 months. Occasional red blood cell transfusions may be required, particularly during febrile illnesses when haemolytic crises are more likely.

## Activity 2.5   Decision-making (p37)

*From what was said in the handover and by your practice supervisor considering issues of gender, ethnicity, and Olufemi's sickle-cell disorder, what about Olufemi is being stigmatised and why do you think he's being stigmatised?*

The racial stereotype of the angry violent young Black man is unfortunately a strong one, and this may dominate the interaction with you and your practice supervisor. He can be stereotyped due to having sickle-cell disease and the racially stereotyped 'drug-seeking behaviour', based on the opiate medication required to manage the pain. In this case, the medication is being assumed to have been requested for reasons of addiction, not pain management. Olufemi is being racialised due to his ethnicity and potentially discriminated against because of this by the individual nurse and the systemic culture of the organisation that perpetuates this. There is evidence that pain management, which is an important part of his nursing care, is not being conducted successfully due to racially based unconscious bias, and poor clinical decision-making due to this by healthcare professionals.

*Olufemi is obviously angry. Why do you think this is?*

His pain is not being managed and he is not being listened to. In previous encounters with healthcare professionals, they may have managed his pain inadequately, with nursing staff not knowing about how to manage his condition appropriately. This could easily have led to his angry behaviour. Think about how you would feel if you were in severe pain, and it was not being managed in a clinical environment that should be able to manage your pain effectively.

*What could you and your practice supervisor do to improve this situation?*

Listen to your patient, particularly when they have a long-term condition and communicate clearly. They may well know more about their condition and how to manage it than you, so work with them. Explain what you are doing as well as why you are doing it. Manage what is obviously his main concern – pain management. Think about why he is behaving in the way he is and look beyond your unconscious bias.

## Activity 2.6   Evidence-based practice and research (p38)

*Find the three determinants of health that the WHO identify as important.*

1.   The social and economic environment.

2.   The physical environment.

3.   The person's individual characteristics and behaviours.

*Find the other seven factors that they consider to determine whether people are healthy or not.*

1.   *Income and social status*

2.   *Education*

3.   *Physical environment*

4.   *Social support networks*

5.   *Genetics*

6.   *Health services*

7.   *Gender*

# Further reading

**Centre for Aging Better** (2022) The state of aging. Summary. Available at: **https://ageing-better. org.uk/sites/default/files/2022-04/The-State-of-Ageing-2022-online.pdf** (accessed 23 July 2022).

This document gives a summary of a comprehensive review of national data on ageing that took place and offers explanations for the changes happening to the older population pre- and during the pandemic.

**Jarrett, S and Tilley, E** (2022) The history of the history of learning disability. *British Journal of Learning Disabilities.*

This article looks at the history of learning disability in society.

**NHS Digital** (2021) Health and Care of people with learning disabilities experimental statistics 2019 to 2020 in *Health and Care of People with Learning Disabilities*. Available at: **https://digital.nhs.uk/data-and-information/publications/statistical/health-and-care-of-people-with-learning-disabilities/experimental-statistics-2019-to-2020#** (accessed 30 May 2022).

This report looks in detail at data and evidence on all aspects of care for people with LDs.

**Phillips, C** (2021) How COVID-19 has exacerbated LGBTQ+ health inequalities. *BMJ*, 372.

This article addresses the inadequate monitoring of health in the LGBTQIA+ community; the data suggest a disproportionate effect of the COVID-19 pandemic and its control measures.

**Royal College of Physicians** (2021) *COVID-19 and Mitigating Impact on Health Inequalities*. Available at: **www.rcplondon.ac.uk/news/covid-19-and-mitigating-impact-health-inequalities** (accessed 6 June 2022).

Examples of how NHS providers have mitigated the impact of COVID-19 on health inequalities.

## Useful websites

Friends, Families and Travellers. Getting a fair deal for Gypsies, Roma, and Travellers:

**www.gypsy-traveller.org/**

This organisation works to end racism and discrimination against Gypsy, Roma, and Traveller people and to protect their right to pursue a nomadic way of life.

ILGA World – The international lesbian, gay, bisexual, trans, and intersex association:

**https://ilga.org/**

Since 1978, ILGA has been committed to equal human rights for rainbow communities and their liberation from all forms of discrimination. They support LGBTQIA+ civil society worldwide through advocacy and research projects and give grassroots movements a voice within international organisations.

National LGBT Research Report:

**www.gov.uk/government/publications/national-lgbt-survey-summary-report**

An analysis of responses to a survey of the experiences of LGBTQIA+ people in British society.

World Health Organization (2008b) *Closing the Gap in a Generation: Health Equity Through Action on the Social Determinants of Health – Final Report of the Commission on Social Determinants of Health.* Geneva: WHO.

**www.who.int/publications/i/item/WHO-IER-CSDH-08.1**

Learning Disability:

**www.learningdisability.co.uk/**

A useful website that has valuable videos from people with learning disabilities and key points of importance when working with people with learning disabilities.

Scottish Learning Disabilities Observatory:

**www.sldo.ac.uk/**

The Observatory has been set up to provide better information about the health and healthcare of people with learning disabilities and people with autism in Scotland in order to inform actions, practice and policy.

The Health Foundation:

**www.health.org.uk**

An independent charity committed to bringing about better health and healthcare for people in the UK. Its organisers believe that good health supports positive social and economic outcomes – both for the individual and society as a whole – understanding the quality of healthcare through in-depth analysis of policy and data.

Runnymede Trust:

**www.runnymedetrust.org**

Runnymede is a charity and the UK's leading independent race equality think tank. They generate intelligence for a multi-ethnic Britain through research, network-building, leading debate, and policy engagement.

UK Health Security Agency:

**www.gov.uk/government/organisations/uk-health-security-agency**

Responsible for protecting every member of every community from the impact of infectious diseases, chemical, biological, radiological, and nuclear incidents, and other health threats.

# Chapter 3

# Diversity, communication, and health literacy

*Marion Hinds and Beverley Brathwaite*

## NMC Future Nurse: Standards of Proficiency for Registered Nurses

This chapter will address the following platforms and proficiencies:

**Platform 1: Being an accountable professional**

1.9 understand the need to base all decisions regarding care and interventions on people's needs and preferences, recognising and addressing any personal and external factors that may unduly influence their decisions.

1.11 communicate effectively using a range of skills and strategies with colleagues and people at all stages of life and with a range of mental, physical, cognitive and behavioural health challenges.

1.14 provide and promote non-discriminatory, person-centred and sensitive care at all times, reflecting on people's values and beliefs, diverse backgrounds, cultural characteristics, language requirements, needs and preferences, taking account of any need for adjustments.

**Platform 2: Promoting health and preventing ill health**

2.7 understand and explain the contribution of social influences, health literacy, individual circumstances, behaviours and lifestyle choices to mental, physical and behavioural health outcomes.

## Chapter aims

After reading this chapter, you will be able to:

- define and explain the key terms 'health literacy' and 'communication';
- understand the relevant theory supporting the concepts of diversity, health literacy and communication, and their application to healthcare practice;

- understand the need for effective communication in order to improve health literacy in diverse groups; and
- apply knowledge and understanding to a range of work-based scenarios exploring communication and health literacy in diverse groups.

# Introduction

## Case study: Bernard Wright

Bernard Wright is a 70-year-old man who lives in a hostel for the homeless with a history of depression. Currently, he is experiencing weight loss, tiredness, and shortness of breath, and has had a persistent cough for the past three months. His symptoms were noticed by Jacob, one of the care workers, who suggested Bernard see the visiting doctor. He was prescribed two types of antibiotics. However, three weeks later, his symptoms have not improved, and he is feeling worse. Codruta, a second-year mental health student nurse on her first community placement, accompanies the community matron, Mabel, to assess Bernard at the hostel. Bernard is very quiet and looks unkempt. When Mabel questions him, his responses are a simple 'yes' or 'no' without any further details given, despite her trying to coax him to respond with more information. When Mabel leaves the room to speak with Jacob, Codruta decides to move closer to Bernard and starts by introducing herself. She asks him if he minds her talking to him; he does not look at her, but replies, 'No'. Codruta starts by asking Bernard to tell her about his life. He is hesitant at first, but slowly tells her that he became homeless after losing his job at a local factory ten years ago. This triggered his depression, and the pandemic only exacerbated this. Bernard continues, saying that he is very worried about his cough, but when he saw the doctor, he felt hurried, and the appointment was very quick. He says that he was given some tablets and does not remember being given any instructions on what to do. Bernard does not like medicines, so he did not take them and felt that he would eventually get better. He also admits that he has some difficulty with reading, writing, and following information given to him, and feels embarrassed about this.

In this chapter, you will develop an understanding of health literacy and effective communication in relation to the care of diverse groups. Health literacy has varied definitions, but they all have the same core elements which describe 'the literacy and numeracy skills that enable individuals to obtain, understand, appraise, and use the information to make decisions and take actions that will have an impact on health status' (Nutbeam and Lloyd, 2020, p159). Throughout this chapter, there will be activities and the application of patient scenarios from all fields of nursing, and this will enable you to appreciate the requirements and subtle differences when caring for patients from these backgrounds. Variations such as language, dialect, and cultural norms are central parts of how diverse groups communicate and interact with healthcare services and must be taken into consideration during all healthcare episodes.

Over the last two decades, there has been a significant change in the demographics of the United Kingdom. The diversity of groups within the population is on the increase, and this trend is set to continue, meaning diversity in healthcare will continue.

For diverse groups, appropriate person-centred communication in all its forms is a key foundation in providing quality care, as well as ensuring the right access to care services. For example, the inability to engage with healthcare professionals due to issues such as limited English language skills, cognitive disability or a nomadic lifestyle, such as those in the Gypsy, Roma, and Traveller (GRT) communities, will negatively impact on the maintenance of optimum health discussed in this chapter.

Literacy is the capability to read, write, speak, listen, and understand written communication to an appropriate level that enables us to function well in society and to make sense of the world in which we live (National Literacy Trust, 2017). Research shows that more than four in ten adults struggle with health content for the public and more than six in ten adults struggle with health content that includes numbers and statistics (NHS Digital, 2021). In a diverse and often marginalised group, such as those belonging to the GRT communities, low literacy levels are commonplace together with a reduced ability to access computer technology (Scadding and Sweeney, 2018).

Health literacy is defined by NHS Digital (2021) as 'a person's ability to understand and use the information to make decisions about their health'. The Nursing and Midwifery Council Standards (NMC, 2018) define health literacy as 'the degree to which individuals can obtain, process, and understand basic health information and services needed to make appropriate health decisions' (p35). Health literacy can be divided into three categories:

1. *Functional health literacy:* This is described as the basic level of reading, writing, numeracy and discussion skills that an individual will need to function effectively in daily life.

2. *Communicative/interactive health literacy:* It is important for individuals to have skills that equip them with the ability to distinguish what information is important and relevant. This will, in turn, help them to make good and effective health decisions.

3. *Critical health literacy:* This is about an individual having greater control over their life by using the skill of critical analysis when sourcing information. This includes areas such as the promotion of health and well-being and the self-management of their own conditions.

Healthcare professionals must recognise the importance of patients having adequate health literacy skills during healthcare interactions (NHS Digital, 2021). During the pandemic, the need for clear health literacy to aid reduced transmission of COVID-19 and the use of the vaccine has been a major priority for healthcare. Effective communication is the cornerstone for all fields of nursing, and is one of the ways in which compassion, sensitivity, and caring can be conveyed in order to promote collaboration and cooperation in the clinical setting (Neale and Sale, 2022).

You will now have knowledge of some key terms that are used when exploring the subject of health literacy. The next section will provide you with information on self-awareness and how it can negatively and positively influence your interactions with patients.

# Self-awareness

The NMC Code (2018b) identifies that prioritising people calling for tolerance and acceptance of others, even if you do not understand their particular way of life, should not affect the care that you provide. As a student nurse, you will need to develop the skills of self-awareness and self-care to know and understand yourself in order to understand and relate to others (van Vilet et al., 2018; Rasheed et al., 2019). Rasheed et al. (2019, p763) identified the importance of self-awareness for nurses. Here is a summary of some of the key points:

Self-awareness enables nurses to recognise their emotional states, thoughts, feelings, biases, strengths, and limitations in general as well as in any given nursing situation. Becoming more self-aware prevents nurses from projecting their personal biases and values onto their patients and others.

Self-awareness does not only include examining one's traits and emotions, but it also includes examining environmental and contextual factors that may influence nurse–patient interactions.

Self-awareness is especially needed for healthcare providers to manage their cognitive, affective, and behavioural self, which helps in improving their caring behaviours.

If you do not understand self-awareness and how you portray yourself, not only can you cause offence to already isolated and marginalised groups, but your ability to develop effective interactions with patients will be limited.

The following scenario provides an example of how life experience and self-awareness can potentially influence a patient admission in the clinical setting.

## Scenario: hospital admission of a service user with a learning disability

Jonas is a third-year learning disability nursing student who has just started a placement on an adult surgical assessment ward. He is working with his practice assessor, Jatinder, who is currently admitting 18-year-old Max, who lives at home. He has autism and is able to make himself understood. Max is accompanied by his sister Kirsty, who says that Max has abdominal pain but that she does not know anything more. Max appears quiet and withdrawn and

*(Continued)*

(Continued)

does not make eye contact; he is also groaning intermittently. Jatinder is finding the situation challenging as there is limited information available and she is becoming frustrated as Max is reluctant to communicate. Jonas is confident in his experience in situations such as this due to his training so far. He also has a younger brother with autism but has never talked to anyone at work about this. He would like to talk to Max but feels reluctant to do so.

As you can see from this scenario, there are a number of aspects to think about in terms of using appropriate and effective communication strategies when caring for Max.

Activity 3.1 now asks you some questions in relation to the scenario about Max.

## Activity 3.1   Reflection

After reading the above scenario, consider the following questions:

- How do you think Max might be feeling?
- Why do you think Jonas is feeling reluctant to intervene, and what should he do in this situation?

*An outline answer can be found at the end of the chapter.*

The next scenario will highlight an example of an interaction between a health professional and a mother and her child from a diverse group. Communication with children and parents will require skills and knowledge of child development and learning ability, as well as any diverse group considerations. For the GRT community challenges include the regular movement of these groups, reduced access to services based on discrimination, and therefore continued and regular access to healthcare services can be sporadic. Read the scenario below, which concerns a health consultation between a Traveller mother, her child, and the diabetes nurse specialist.

## Scenario: health consultation with a mother and child

Selina is a 9-year-old girl who was diagnosed with type 1 diabetes during the pandemic. Her family are Travellers, and they tend to move around the country quite frequently. Since this diagnosis, the family have remained in the local area. Selina lives with her mother, father, and two brothers in a mobile home. She is having a consultation with Lucia, the diabetes nurse specialist, regarding the stabilisation of her condition. There have been ongoing challenges in the management of her blood glucose levels. Selina attends the local primary school, and she is very sociable and energetic. Selina has attended the appointment with her mother, who is very anxious about this meeting, and keeps stating that she 'does not know why this has happened to Selina'. Lucia is aware from previous encounters that Selina's mother has only recently come around to accepting her daughter's condition. More recently, Selina has been complaining that she is very tired.

In situations such as those described above, communication can be hindered by health beliefs that can be held by the parties involved. This calls for sensitivity by the nurse towards both Selina and her mother in order to facilitate effective person-centred care. However, always remember that your patient has individual needs and values.

Activity 3.2 asks you to think about the situation presented in the above scenario about Selina.

## Activity 3.2   Communication and decision-making

- What issues concerning Selina and her health need to be considered?
- What can be done to help Selina's mother cope better with the current situation?

*An outline answer can be found at the end of the chapter.*

Continuing with the importance of communication between healthcare professionals and patients, the following case study provides a stark illustration of the implications of poor health literacy and communication breakdown, the circumstances of which involved a young mother, a father, and their new-born baby.

## Case study: significant failure of communication

In July 2009, a 21-year-old woman gave birth to a healthy baby boy at a local general hospital. The parents were Tamil refugees from Sri Lanka and the mother spoke only a few words of English. Two days later, mother and baby were discharged from the hospital in the early afternoon but could not leave until approximately eight hours later, when the father and a friend who spoke better English were coming to collect them. By this time, the baby was continuously crying; however, the mother was told by the midwives that this was normal behaviour in new-borns. The father had asked if mother and baby could remain in hospital another two days, when he would be off work and more able to assist at home, but was told this was not possible. When the father and friend arrived, the friend questioned if the

*(Continued)*

(Continued)

discharge should go ahead as the baby was crying, but was told it was normal. The friend and parents took the baby to the car and again returned to ask if a doctor could look at the baby, but were told again that crying was normal. They were advised that if anything was wrong, they could bring the baby back. The community midwife arrived at 12.40 p.m. the next day at the couple's home and found the baby 'pale, lethargic, and not interested in feeding' (Dyer, 2018, p1). The baby had not been fed since more than 15 hours earlier and there was no milk formula in the house. An ambulance was called; however, the baby 'was in a hypoglycaemic state' (Dyer, 2018, p1), which caused severe, catastrophic brain injuries.

The child now has cerebral palsy and severe physical and cognitive impairment. Failings were found in terms of poor communication engagement with the mother due to language barriers. Unfortunately, this was a poor discharge as opportunities for a safe discharge outcome, such as the use of an interpreter to facilitate better communication with the mother, were missed. The case was taken to court and the judge ruled that if the baby had been checked before the family left the hospital, the outcome would have been avoided. It was acknowledged that the mother had attempted to voice her concerns, but due to the language barrier she could not make herself understood. As such, no information had been provided to the parents in relation to the necessity of feeding their new-born baby. Additionally, the provision of information from staff that could be easily understood by the parents was not demonstrated in this tragic case.

As the above case study clearly demonstrates, skilled engagement with individuals from diverse backgrounds requires the consideration of certain nuances, terminology, and norms which the healthcare professional may not know about. It is therefore necessary that, as a student nurse, you develop effective, purposeful, person-centred communication skills to successfully perform in your current and future role as a registered nurse. Another key component of this process is the ability to facilitate an appropriate level of engagement with the patient in order to enable a responsive and meaningful therapeutic relationship. Diverse groups with linguistic needs must be recognised and appropriate care delivered (Bonakdar et al., 2022). They need to trust the healthcare professional to care for them. Effective communication is clearly linked to patient safety (Fuchshuber and Greif, 2022).

From reading this chapter so far, you will have an idea of the necessity for good communication skills and what can happen if this does not occur. The next section will discuss in more detail communication and health literacy as applied to diverse groups.

# Communication and health literacy in diverse groups

Evidence consistently finds that effective communication is vital to the safe delivery of care and even more so in marginalised communities (Simonovich et al., 2021; Kwame and Petrucka, 2021).

Before continuing to read the rest of the chapter, take some time to complete Activity 3.3.

## Activity 3.3    Research and reflection

Write down your own definition of the word 'communication' and the different types you can find.

Look up two definitions of the word 'communication'. What are the similarities and in what ways do they differ?

What strategies would you use in order to communicate with someone who did not share the same language as you?

*There is no model answer at the end of the chapter as this is based on your own reflections; however, the next section provides some outline answers to the questions.*

Having thought about the issues raised in Activity 3.3, it is apparent that, as a nurse, communication is possibly the most important skill that is required when dealing with patients. The process involves the whole being and is at the heart of the delivery of quality nursing care. It is the foundation upon which we develop and maintain relationships, and there are certain ethical, legal, and professional implications for nurses. However, communication is of no use if the recipient is unable to understand and act upon the information being given. As human beings, we each communicate in a number of ways and by various methods. Good communication will depend upon the skill of the health professional to deliver a clear message to the patient (Neale and Sale, 2022).

Communication may be simply defined as the interactive passage or passing of information between parties – sender and receiver – using means such as writing, speaking or the use of a common sign system of behaviour (Ali, 2017). More recently, the use of online platforms has become increasingly popular, especially during the pandemic out of necessity, which adds to both the ease and complexity of communicating.

However, if you think about the process of communication, you will appreciate that it can be fraught with difficulty, as once something is said it cannot be taken back; in other words, it is irreversible. Another definition is that communication is the 'imparting or exchanging of information by speaking, writing, or using some other medium' (Lexico, 2019a). You may find that when exploring the definition of the word 'communication', there are more similarities than differences. Examples of similarities may include:

- The process involves more than one person, and those involved will take on the role of sender or receiver, and these roles can interchange during the communication interaction.

- Communication is also dependent upon the context or circumstances in which the process takes place.
- An integral part of the process is that those involved will understand the messages being passed between each other.
- There are numerous influences that can enhance and disrupt the communication process.
- The purpose of communication models is to explain the complexity of communication theory.

A key difference in communication definitions may be found in the wording used to describe the term. There are also subtle differences in the components that make up theoretical models such as the transactional model of communication, which is described on pp58–59.

Groups tend to share common verbal and non-verbal ways in which initial greetings are made when meeting with others (e.g. the spoken word or the use of body language, such as a handshake, nod, or smile). Each individual will attach specific meaning to these responses.

As a student, you need to be mindful of individual patient behaviour during the health and illness continuum. The presentation and experience of signs and symptoms in areas such as pain and anxiety can alter the communication process (Bloomfield and Pegram, 2015). The NMC (2018b) makes clear that, as a nurse, you are to

*provide and promote non-discriminatory, person-centred, and sensitive care at all times, reflecting on people's values and beliefs, diverse backgrounds, cultural characteristics, language requirements, needs and preferences, taking account of any need for adjustments.*

(p9)

Communication with patients can be problematic for a number of reasons, the most important being an assumption that the information delivered is understood and will be appropriately acted upon. For diverse and often vulnerable groups, there will be additional unique differences, such as age, culture, linguistic needs, income, socio-economic position, and cognitive ability, and these can adversely impact upon their access and engagement with healthcare services. The global emergence of health literacy as a concept is borne out of this and the recognition that health literacy is a significant determinant of health status (WHO, 2013).

Health literacy is relevant during all stages of the life continuum, and a lack of key literate skills will negatively impact an individual's life from childhood to adulthood. Many people function adequately with low literacy skills and illiteracy and never disclose their limitations. There is no way to distinguish if a person has a low level of literacy, and educational achievement is not a reliable indicator. There is a link between shame, stigma, and health literacy, which leads to poorer health outcomes (Mackert et al., 2019). This topic was identified at the beginning of this chapter in the case study about Bernard Wright.

As a nurse, you need to ensure that you deal sensitively with issues of literacy. Signs of low literacy include the patient asking very few or no questions, non-compliance with medications, and the inability to provide a coherent history of complaints and complete forms. In addition to regularly missed appointments, the identification of medications by sight (rather than reading labels) and being unable to explain their prescribed medications.

A report published by the National Literacy Trust confirmed that *people with low levels of literacy are more likely to live in deprived communities, be financially worse off, and have poorer health* (Gilbert et al., 2018, p3). Literacy has an impact upon people's ability to access and use information. This further confirms the need to address the health literacy needs of diverse populations.

Another key aspect of terminology when considering health literacy is mental health literacy (MHL), which is defined as the *knowledge and beliefs about mental disorders which aid their recognition, management or prevention* (Jorm et al., 1997). It is possible to conclude that if an individual experiences life-affecting psychological symptoms, they will attempt to manage the symptoms. Therefore, symptom management strategies, such as seeking support from family and friends, will be influenced by an individual's own level of mental health literacy (Nutbeam and Muscat, 2020).

Public Health England identifies that policymakers at the local and government level must collaborate with the health and social care sectors, including schools, employers, and adult education services, to address the health literacy agenda (PHE, 2015).

In the next scenario about Miles, you will be able to explore the concept of mental health literacy further.

## Scenario: mental health literacy

Miles is a 24-year-old Black British Caribbean man who was diagnosed with schizophrenia three years previously. Initially, he was not accepting of his condition, and this led to his non-compliance with prescribed medication. He was admitted to an acute mental health ward for assessment and further management. He is now stabilised and lives in social housing accommodation, and Imran is his assigned key worker. Miles has close ties with his mother and father and visits them daily, often staying over if he does not feel like going home. His mother is very involved with his condition and ongoing care. One evening while he is watching television, his mother notices a plaster on his arm and asks him what has happened. Miles tells her that he received a call earlier in the day to attend an appointment with Basil, the mental health nurse, and a blood test was taken. Miles has no idea why. His mother is very upset that he is unable to give her any further information and plans to call Basil the next day to find out what is going on.

Take time to reflect on what you have read so far on health and mental health literacy before continuing with Activity 3.4.

## Activity 3.4    Reflection and critical thinking

- What do you consider are the issues with Miles?
- What do you think could be done to help Miles?
- What information would you give to Miles's mother?

*An outline answer can be found at the end of the chapter.*

The issue of mental health literacy is one of growing importance given the increase in individuals experiencing mental health problems in society. The key aim of the government's position on mental health is to achieve equality and combat discrimination for individuals and groups experiencing mental health difficulties. Disparities have been identified in the ability to access services among varied ethnic groups, which will have a negative outcome on overall well-being (GOV.UK, 2019). A study carried out by Memon et al. (2016) on perceived barriers to accessing mental health services by various ethnicities in the south of England concluded there were a number of key areas that required attention. The *inability to recognise and accept mental health problems* was cited as a key issue (p1). Language barriers and poor communication were factors that affected relationships between the parties involved. Additionally, men were found to be a *hard-to-reach group* and *were more reluctant to seek help and felt excluded* from services (p7). The study also identified that the responsiveness of services to the diverse needs of various ethnic group service users was limited.

In the next section, we will look at the theoretical basis of a specific communication model and types of communication, such as non-verbal and interpersonal, as well as the use of interpreter services.

# The transactional model of communication

A knowledge-based foundation of communication theory is important for effective nursing practice. The use of a communication model will provide information on the stages of the process and is often graphically represented. However, while this will detail the different aspects, it may not provide the reader with a conscious idea of the multiple complexities involved during the process.

The transactional model of communication developed by Wood in 2004 considers the fact that numerous channels of communication exist during face-to-face interactions. The model also proposes that those involved both send and receive messages simultaneously and are identified as *communicators*. Wood (2004) defines communication as a *systemic process in which people interact with and through symbols to create and interpret meanings* (p503). The term 'symbol' in this context is pertinent as it denotes a meaning that will vary between people. The model is one that is easily applied to communication with diverse groups as it incorporates how the areas of social, relational, and cultural context make up and influence our communication interactions. It is recognised that outside or external interference, known as noise, as well as internal dialogue, will have an effect on the interaction. External noise, for example, may include a patient pressing a call bell in another area of the ward or a telephone ringing. Internal noise might involve the subjective feeling of anger or tiredness in either participant during the communication process.

The model theorises that during this constant flow of verbal and non-verbal messages that pass back and forth between those involved, we are able to construct and revise our communication during the encounter based upon the messages received. The channels of communication will include nuances such as body angle, presentation, and tone of voice (Pavord and Donnelly, 2015). The reaction of each participant during the communication episode will depend upon factors such as cultural beliefs, previous experience, attitude and background.

It is impossible not to communicate, and, as a student nurse, you must develop the skills to take note, interpret, and understand the information provided by the patient. McCarthy et al. (2013) conducted a study among undergraduate student nurses that explored the issues faced when communicating with patients who did not share the same first language. A number of concerns were raised about the student's ability to perform an accurate and comprehensive patient assessment, the effective use of translator services, and the interpretation of non-verbal cues. If you consider the assessment process, for example, it is important to develop a rapport with the patient; if not, this can result in a lack of information that can have a detrimental effect on health outcomes. This further reinforces the complexity and challenge of developing sound communication strategies with others in our care.

A study conducted by Norouzinia et al. (2016) on communication barriers identified that reluctance by nurses to communicate was highlighted by patients as one of the most frequent complaints. The study concluded that the best way to achieve patient satisfaction was through effective and appropriate communication. There can be barriers to communication due to being non-English-speaking, cultural differences in communication causing a lack of understanding, low literacy levels, and health beliefs negatively influencing the hospital experience (Zegers and Auron, 2022).

# Verbal communication

The NMC (2018c) makes clear the requirement of a nurse or midwife to:

*communicate effectively using a range of skills and strategies with colleagues and people at all stages of life and with a range of mental, physical, cognitive and behavioural health challenges.*

(p1)

*provide and promote non-discriminatory, person-centred and sensitive care at all times, reflecting on people's values and beliefs, diverse backgrounds, cultural characteristics, language requirements, needs and preferences, taking account of any need for adjustments.*

(p1)

Verbal communication is the use of the spoken word to participate in a mutual exchange with another. The purpose of this process is to convey and impart information, and will involve attention to the language, dialect, and local variations in use by the patient. It would be unreasonable to expect you, as a student, to be familiar with every aspect of verbal communication style in respect of your patient. However, to purposefully engage with patients, there must be some development of meaningful exchange in order to encourage open dialogue and trust. Argyle et al. (1970) deduced that during a face-to-face interaction, only 7 per cent of a message is made up of words; 55 per cent is body language, with tone, syntax, and tempo making up the remaining 38 per cent. Given that such a small percentage is focused upon the verbal transmission of information, this demonstrates the significant relevance of non-verbal communication. As good practice, try to remember this fact when you next interact with someone whose first language is not English.

# The use of interpreter services

When communicating with individuals who have limited or no understanding of the English language, every effort must be made to secure the services of an interpreter. LanguageLine is a telephone interpretation service that is most frequently used in the UK. If this is not available, then the physical presence of an interpreter has to be employed in order to facilitate an appropriate level of dialogue (Bloomfield and Pegram, 2015). Assistance from a family member or friend should not be considered unless there is no alternative option, it is an emergency situation, or at the patient's request. This must not be normal practice as there is the possibility of passing inaccurate or false information to or on behalf of the patient; in addition, there may be safeguarding implications (Pavord and Donnelly, 2015). The potential to cause harm and compromise safety is increased if there is a mistranslation, a breakdown in communication, or no communication at all (Al Shamsi et al., 2020).

The environment where the communication is to take place should be quiet, away from any disturbances, and the process should not be rushed. The participants should consist only of those who are directly involved, and seating should be arranged in a way that is inclusive and allows for direct communication with the patient, interpreter, and health professional. The health professional must check with the patient as to how they would like to be addressed and introductions made so that the patient is aware of the roles of those present, as well as the purpose of the communication. Speech should be appropriately pitched and paced when speaking to the patient, without the use of complex terminology or jargon, to allow for easy interpretation. If possible, written information should be provided in the patient's first language, and the use of pictures, signs, and symbols can be used to further enhance the patient's understanding. Information provided to the patient should be repeated as often as necessary during the communication process.

Burnham et al. (2008) developed the acronym 'social grraacceess' to assist professionals in the development of their self-awareness skills when working with a range of differences in individuals. As a student, it is recommended that as good practice, you use reflection to develop your knowledge and understanding. Try to think about each of the concepts listed below when you come into contact with patients:

- **G**ender
- **R**ace
- **R**eligion
- **A**ge
- **A**bility
- **C**lass
- **C**ulture
- **E**thnicity
- **E**ducation
- **S**exuality
- **S**pirituality

Before reading further, complete Activity 3.5, which asks you to consider these terms in more detail.

## Activity 3.5   Research and critical thinking

Access relevant resources to find a definition and make your own notes on each of the terms in the above acronym, 'social grraacceess'.

*Definitions for each can be found in the content of this book so will not be provided as an answer at the end of the chapter.*

The previous section explored a communication model, verbal communication, and the use of interpreter services. You should now have a better understanding of the relevance of these components in promoting positive patient–nurse interactions.

The next part of this chapter will examine the components of non-verbal communication, which is necessary given that the majority of our communication is conducted through non-verbal means.

# Interpersonal communication

The 'interpersonal nature of communication' gives specific focus to the way in which two or more individuals or groups are involved and *behave towards and feel about one another* (Bach and Grant, 2015, p14). As a student, you will be involved with patients in varied settings, such as the patient's home, clinic, and the ward, and many issues will require consideration during these interactions. Interpersonal skills are considered a sound basis for professional practice and the development of a patient-centred relationship based upon trust, respect, compassion and understanding (Bloomfield and Pegram, 2015).

# Non-verbal communication

Non-verbal communication is that which is without words, or the use of wordless cues and features such as touch, eye contact, proximity, and head movement. Use of body language, posture, odour, and facial expressions are considered non-verbal expressions of communication (Pavord and Donnelly, 2015). It is important to bear in mind that non-verbal communication is just as powerful as other forms, if not more so, as profound meaning can be transmitted by gestures and even silence (Ali, 2018). In terms of diverse groups, this form of communication can prove challenging, and this is because, as nurses, we may not be conversant with certain cultural expressions, which can lead to misunderstandings in our dealings with patients from diverse groups in our care. Nurses must also be aware of their body language; for example, a nurse who appears to be very busy may be perceived by the patient as unapproachable, so care may be delayed, which may result in negative consequences.

Good listening skills demonstrate that you are interested in those to whom you are relating, and at times can be hard to achieve. When listening, you should give the speaker your undivided attention, focus on the words being spoken, and try not to interrupt. In the delivery of nursing care, it is important that you ask for clarification if there is something said that you do not understand – ask the patient or service user for clarification. It is necessary that you maintain an open mind and try not to stereotype so that you can be receptive to, for example, older patients and LGBTQIA+ service users.

Eye contact or gaze can be an indication of the level of attention being paid to the speaker, and vice versa, and plays a vital role in social interactions (Sibiya, 2018).

Imagine if you were speaking with someone and their gaze was elsewhere – your cultural background would play a key part in your interpretation of the situation. In Western society, it is polite to give eye contact and a sign that you may have something to hide if you do not. In West African culture, it is considered a sign of disrespect for young people to directly gaze into the eyes of an older person (elder) (Fafunwa, 2018). Knowledge or discussion with the patient or service user will be necessary so as not to mistakenly cause any offence.

The use of touch during communication enhances the encounter, but only when appropriate (e.g. in the delivery of physical care). In some circumstances, such as communicating bad news, while touch might seem appropriate, it might not be to the recipient (Bagci and Cinar Yucel, 2020). Touch is linked to the demonstration of empathy, and offers a physical connection to another, but must be used with caution. Each communication encounter with individuals from diverse groups is unique. If the nurse has any doubts about the appropriateness of touch, it is better to withhold this gesture until certain, so as not to cause any offence. In line with touch is the proximity of one individual to another, also known as personal space. Situations will differ, and if we are engaged in personal care activities or supporting a patient where close distance is necessary, understanding that this might be uncomfortable or disagreeable to some individuals is necessary. In situations such as these, attention must be paid to the non-verbal responses a patient or service user may convey.

Body language is a powerful tool and aids the communication process. People communicate continuously; even our type of dress or the way we sit or position ourselves will send a message to others. Aspects such as age, gender, and social position can influence the communication process in a positive or negative manner.

Consider the scenario in Activity 3.6, which you may well encounter at some stage in your practice. This provides a typical example of the need to recognise and, insofar as possible, accurately interpret a patient's body language during interactions.

## Activity 3.6   Communication and reflection

Imagine that yourself and another nurse are in the process of turning a patient who is bed-bound and speaks limited English. You notice that the patient has her eyes closed; she is grimacing and squeezing your hand.

- What are your thoughts about how the patient might be feeling?
- Imagine the same scenario, but this time the patient has her eyes open and is smiling at you.
- What are your thoughts now about how the patient might be feeling?

*An outline answer is provided at the end of the chapter.*

The chapter will continue by discussing two further areas of the communication process, namely intrapersonal communication and paralanguage.

# Intrapersonal communication

Intrapersonal communication requires us to know ourselves and is the form of communication that takes place within us on a constant basis (Welch, 2022). This form of internal dialogue enables us to think, feel, and recollect on certain narratives and enables learning to take place. Reflection is a tool that enables us to break down and examine situations and experiences that are encountered within and outside of practice. As nurses, reflection is a key component of the learning process, and according to Price (2017), *reflective practice is at the centre of nursing* (p53). To engage in a process of self-reflection allows for professional growth and development in terms of understanding who we are as well as those around us.

# Paralanguage

Paralanguage is that which refers to accent, speed of the spoken word, tone, and pitch, which have considerable negative and positive implications when communicating with diverse groups. Put simply, it is the way in which we pitch our tone and speak with particular emphasis upon certain words, which will change the meaning of the sentence. The delivery of a simple sentence can cause a breakdown in the nurse–patient relationship, as well as causing distress and anxiety to the patient. As explained by Richardson (2017), *paralanguage makes clear what the meaning is* (p30). It is an attempt to 'understand the mood or emotional state of the person' (p30). However, paralanguage in certain groups may be misunderstood and lead to stereotyping and bias. An example of this is the *angry Black woman*, as discussed by Waldron (2019), who, against the backdrop of mental health issues, explores the negativity surrounding personal descriptors used to explain behaviour apparently exhibited by Black women. Terms such as 'aggressive', 'ignorant', 'hostile', and 'ill-tempered' do nothing to dispel the myths that further compound the negative stereotyping towards them. What you can do depending upon the given situation is appreciate the range of emotions during the communication process, such as anger, fear, sadness, anxiety, grief, and shame. Allow sufficient time for the patient to convey their feelings.

Many barriers exist that can hinder the development of effective communication during the nurse–patient relationship. The next section will provide a summary of those barriers associated with communication among diverse groups, some of which have been highlighted throughout this chapter.

# Communication barriers and diverse groups

Activity 3.7 asks you to think about possible barriers to the communication process.

---

## Activity 3.7   Reflection

Make a list of as many communication barriers that you can think of and/or those you may have observed in clinical practice.

You may find that the barriers can be separated into categories such as nurse, patient, or environmental-related factors.

Suggest one solution for each barrier example you have listed.

*There is no outline answer at the end of the chapter, but some possible answers to the questions above are provided in the next section.*

---

As identified in your reading so far, communication with diverse groups within the UK population is worthy of in-depth consideration given the complexities that may arise. Coupled with this are the potential barriers that may be encountered during the communication process, some of which are listed below.

## Professional barriers

These include aspects such as limited resources, lack of time, increased workload capacity, staff conflict, and fatigue, all of which can affect the communication process. The use of masks during the pandemic has brought its own challenges with communication, as reduced facial expression, the ability to read lips, and the reduced sound caused by mask-wearing impacted communication, but more so for patients with a learning disability (LD), mental health problems, and the elderly.

## Relationship dynamics

The importance of the dynamics of the people involved in the communication process must not be underestimated, and will include the patient, nurse, and any other member of the MDT. A lack of understanding will lead to poor patient engagement and comprehension. Previous poor experience with healthcare professionals will impact on subsequent interactions, which can negatively influence patient understanding, following healthcare advice. This is more common for those from Black and Asian ethnic groups, migrant communities, patients with LDs, mental health concerns, and disabilities than for the general population (Latif et al., 2018).

## Chapter summary

After reading this chapter, you should now have a good understanding of the importance of effective communication to improve health literacy in diverse groups. The vulnerability of such groups makes them more susceptible to less than adequate healthcare provision and poorer access. Health literacy remains a vast field of study, largely due to the recognition that patient and service user limitations in this area will impact negatively on health outcomes and life span. With the advent of an increasingly diverse group population and advances in healthcare, it is vital that we, as health professionals, continue to address the issues involving communication and health literacy. This will in turn narrow the gap and facilitate better access to services. Nurses must continually develop and maintain their communication skills to encompass all areas of verbal and non-verbal communication. This will provide quality individualised person-centred care that is both relevant and applicable to the diverse groups living in today's society.

## Activities: brief outline answers

### Activity 3.1    Reflection (p52)

Max may well be feeling very scared, possibly stressed, as he is not in his normal environment, and he is with staff who are not familiar to him. Added to this is the physiological symptom of pain, which is likely to cause increased anxiety and fear of what will happen. It is important that the way in which Max is expressing himself, verbally and non-verbally, is taken into account. This may be more pronounced in persons with a learning disability. There is a possibility that Max might identify and interact better with Jonas as he is a male nurse. Information will need to be obtained from as many sources as possible. This will enable staff to build a picture of Max's usual behaviour; however, in the case study, it would appear that information is limited. Therefore, Kirsty, Jonas, and Jatinder need to think of appropriate ways in which to engage with Max. Aspects such as the tone of voice, body proximity, touch, language, and the use of friendly words that Max will understand can be helpful. Contact with a family member, friend, or significant other will also alleviate fear and bring some normalisation to the situation for Max, if contact is possible and appropriate. If available, the learning disability liaison nurse can provide expert advice. This role has been proven to have achieved positive outcomes for persons with learning disabilities admitted to hospital (Tuffrey-Wijne et al., 2013). While Jonas has personal experience of learning disability, this is a work environment, and he might be feeling that as a student he is there to learn rather than to share his knowledge. It is recommended that he should speak with Jatinder and offer some suggestions. Jonas might also wish to tell Jatinder of his brother's condition if he feels comfortable enough to do so.

### Activity 3.2    Communication and decision-making (p53)

In this scenario, Selina could be anxious and frightened due to her condition, and this will be increased by her mother's apparent refusal to accept the situation. It is likely that she might be feeling ill at ease despite having met Lucia previously. Schooling and social environment will impact upon Selina's understanding; however, at this age, it is likely that she will be asking questions, and Lucia must work to engage her in the discussion to ascertain her thoughts and feelings (Bach and Grant, 2015). The use of graphic materials will help to aid Selina's knowledge and promote participation. At this age, it is likely that Selina may be heavily influenced by her mother's behaviour. Therefore, in order to achieve a positive outcome to the meeting, it will be necessary to develop a productive relationship with Selina's mother. It will then be possible to explore her lack of acceptance and the reasons for this. Lucia will need to convey respect for the cultural background and appreciate the strongly held beliefs the mother might have. One way of approaching this is to ask the mother for more information about her health beliefs. The use of various communication techniques, such as allowing both Selina and her mother the opportunity to speak without interruption and not using jargon, will assist in reducing barriers. Lucia will also need to identify whether there are any illiteracy problems that are hindering the understanding of Selina or her mother. This will also demonstrate that Lucia is a collaborative partner in healthcare to work with, not against. Contact with other health professionals, such as the general practitioner (GP) and the consultant in charge of Selina's case, as well as the school, will be other sources of relevant information. As Selina is showing the physical symptoms of tiredness, this will also require investigation as the diabetes might not be well controlled. If Lucia has any concerns about the vulnerability of Selina in the current situation, a safeguarding referral might be appropriate. Safeguarding is about the right of individuals to be safe from harm; in relation to children, one of the key areas is the prevention of impairment of children's health or development. The NMC (2018a) makes clear that we all have a role to play in safeguarding vulnerable adults and children in society. This would have to be discussed with Selina's parents so that they are fully informed and understand the reasons for this course of action, if deemed necessary.

## Activity 3.4  Reflection and critical thinking (p58)

It is apparent from the scenario that Miles possesses some mental health literacy skills in terms of the continued treatment of his condition. There is significant relevance attached to the level of engagement and understanding of an individual's health condition. It is important to work with Miles by inviting him to a meeting to find out how much he does know about his schizophrenia and the treatment he is receiving. As mentioned earlier in the chapter, self-awareness is a key factor during collaboration with patients and service users. Recognition of how we, as healthcare professionals, present ourselves to others can have the potential to adversely affect the therapeutic relationship. The presence of Imran as an advocate is a necessary advantage, ensuring that Miles's autonomy is protected, and also as an intermediary if required. During the meeting, the language used, and the information provided must be appropriate and acceptable to Miles, otherwise there will be no beneficial outcome. There may be several reasons why Miles has minimal health literacy skills; as identified in this chapter, these could range from poor literacy skills to ethnicity and gender. However, it could be the case that Miles is not motivated to engage with healthcare services. Alternatively, he may not want to inform his mother of the reason for the blood sample, or it might be that he has other support networks with whom he feels more comfortable discussing aspects of his health. It should be remembered that in terms of healthcare communication, not all individuals wish to have in-depth discussion about their conditions. As nurses, we need to recognise and gauge the patient or service user's requirements, and information should be tailored accordingly. The concern expressed by Miles's mother is to be expected; however, as an adult with full mental capacity, he is not compelled to talk to anyone about his health status unless he chooses to do so. It may be necessary for a member of the healthcare team to speak with Miles's mother to explain the relevance of privacy and confidentiality in terms of the disclosure of information that has not been consented to. The fact that Miles is willing to attend appointments is a positive factor in the management of his ongoing treatment.

## Activity 3.6  Communication and reflection (p63)

From this scenario, it may be surmised that in the first context, the patient could be confused, frightened, or in pain. In the second, it could be that the patient is comfortable and willing to be turned and is using her facial expression to communicate this to the nurse. It takes practice and experience to accurately interpret non-verbal communication, but it is a necessary skill that can be developed. We can conclude that in terms of non-verbal communication, facial expression is linked to certain emotions and is a powerful tool with which to communicate with others.

# Further reading

**Centers for Disease Control and Prevention (CDC) (2020)** *Health Literacy. Older Adults.* Available at: **www.cdc.gov/healthliteracy/developmaterials/audiences/olderadults/index.html** (accessed 3 October 2022).

The CDC is American, however this page provides tools and resources to help public health professionals improve their communication with older adults by focusing on health literacy issues.

**Marler, H and Ditton, A** (2021) 'I'm smiling back at you': exploring the impact of mask wearing on communication in healthcare. *International Journal of Language & Communication Disorders,* 56(1): 205–14.

An article that is a reminder of wearing a mask and communication through the pandemic. Still relevant as many people are still masking due to the ongoing pandemic, while the wearing of face masks in the hospital setting still continues in some settings and circumstances.

**World Health Organization (WHO)** (2013) *Health Literacy: The Solid Facts.* Available at: **www.euro. who.int/__data/assets/pdf_file/0008/190655/e96854.pdf** (accessed 2 October 2022).

An informative document that contains evidence in support of the need for a 'whole of society' approach to this concept.

**Zegers, C and Auron, M** (2022) Addressing the Challenges of Cross-Cultural Communication. *Medical Clinics,* 106(4): 577–88.

A journal article that looks at healthcare workers and communicating across multiple cultures.

# Useful websites

## Health literacy

NHS Digital Service Manual:

**https://service-manual.nhs.uk/content/health-literacy**

NHS services are for everyone. But many adults in the UK have low health literacy skills. This means they struggle to read and understand medical content intended for the public.

Health Literacy Place:

**www.healthliteracyplace.org.uk**

A Scottish-based resource website that provides information on aspects related to health literacy.

# Chapter 4　Cultural competency

### Marion Hinds and Mariama Seray-Wurie

## NMC Future Nurse: Standards of Proficiency for Registered Nurses

This chapter will address the following platforms and proficiencies:

### Platform 1: Being an accountable professional

1.14　provide and promote non-discriminatory, person-centred, and sensitive care at all times, reflecting on people's values and beliefs, diverse backgrounds, cultural characteristics, language requirements, needs and preferences, taking account of any need for adjustments.

### Platform 3: Assessing needs and planning care

3.4　understand and apply a person-centred approach to nursing care, demonstrating shared assessment, planning, decision-making and goal setting when working with people, their families, communities and populations of all ages.

## Chapter aims

After reading this chapter, you will be able to:

- discuss the key terms 'culture', 'competence', and 'cultural competence' and their relevance to nursing practice;
- gain insight into the relevant theory supporting the concepts of culture, competence and cultural competency, and their application to healthcare practice;
- appreciate the need for nurses to be culturally competent in healthcare settings;
- apply knowledge and understanding to a range of work-based scenarios exploring cultural competence among patients, clients, and service users.

# Introduction

## Case study: nurse who force-fed her baby

In 2011, a Ghanaian nurse was found guilty of causing or allowing the death of her 10-month-old baby by force-feeding her liquidised food from small, spouted china jugs over a number of months (Guardian Press Association, 2011). Force-feeding involved placing the spout into the child's mouth, effectively preventing her from being able to close her mouth if she did not want any more food. The post-mortem examination concluded that pneumonia caused by foods, including meat and cereals, present in her lungs was the cause of death. The mother was described as being obsessed with her baby's weight and used this method of feeding when weaning her. She admitted that her baby often vomited after feeding but that she did not worry because her other children had done the same. It was claimed that the defendant had previously been warned by doctors and social workers about the dangers of this practice but ignored the advice (Guardian Press Association, 2011). She stated during the trial that this type of feeding was widely used and was the way she and her siblings were fed by their mother in Ghana, and that she had done nothing to hurt her child. During the court proceedings, it was acknowledged that a death of this type, although rare, was a potential outcome of force-feeding. The prosecution stated, 'The mother, she is a nurse, and that involves a degree of extra insight. An ordinary mother would think twice or more before using a jug to pour food into the mouth of a child' (Guardian Press Association, 2011). The Chair of the Safeguarding Children Board confirmed that steps were being taken to provide better information nationally about this practice. The mother was subsequently convicted and sentenced to three years' imprisonment (Guardian Press Association, 2011). Her name was also permanently removed from the NMC register as her fitness to practice was found to be impaired by the nature of this conviction (NMC, 2012).

Culture is complex, as you may now appreciate after reading through the case study above and the previous chapters in this book. Culture is made up of many elements; some are clear to see, while others are not. The concept is generally viewed as shared notions, such as values, practices, beliefs, and traditions that are held by group members who identify as the same culture. These characteristics are in many cases strongly held, and are often passed on through generations, and can therefore be deeply rooted.

The purpose of this chapter is to explore the origin of cultural competency; the key terms 'culture', 'competence', and 'cultural competency', and key theories to develop cultural competence, will be discussed. The chapter will also examine the relevance of nursing models and frameworks and their application in order to develop the knowledge, skills, and attitude relevant to a holistic plan of care that incorporates a patient's cultural identity. A variety of activities and scenarios will guide you to link theory to practice and further develop an understanding of your own cultural competency.

Returning to the case study of the mother who force-fed her baby, it can be seen that one's culture encompasses both health and illness and can strongly influence areas of an individual's life. This includes aspects such as the timing when medical assistance is sought when unwell (Giger and Davidhizar, 2002) and the level of engagement that your patient will maintain in terms of recommended treatment regimes. Certain actions may be taken by the individual that are seen to be the 'right way of doing things', despite the possibility of causing harm. The case study highlights specific areas of consideration that add to the challenges when understanding the practices of people from different cultures. Three areas are worth discussing in relation to the case study:

1.  *Mother's culture:* As already highlighted, culture is complex, and the mother will have been strongly influenced by her upbringing and the commonly held beliefs and values of her background. In the case study, it is evident that the mother was following traditional feeding practices that were carried on through generations in her family. The strength of these beliefs was demonstrated by evidence in court documents that showed she had been advised against the practice of force-feeding her baby by health and social professionals. What must also be taken into account is that in her experience, she had fed her older children in the same way and came to the conclusion that as no harm had come to them, there was nothing untoward with continuing the practice. When conflict or discord occurs between people who hold differing cultural 'values, beliefs, assumptions, and expectations of care', a culture or cultural clash is said to exist (Srivastava, 2003, p35). This clearly demonstrates the strong influence of one's cultural background.

2.  *Professional nursing culture:* From a professional perspective, the mother was a registered nurse, and this would imply that she possessed a specific level of knowledge and skill in terms of health and illness. As a nurse, you are accountable in practice to ensure patient safety and that no harm comes to those in your care (NMC, 2018a). A fundamental part of this is the use of evidence-based interventions. The fact that the individual carried out this practice in her role as a mother does not condone her actions – hence the criminal charges laid against her. This is a challenging point of contention as the mother did not perceive herself as inflicting deliberate harm on her child.

3.  *British culture:* In Western society, the biomedical model of healthcare is the most dominant. Its basis lies in the scientific and biological factors of illness and disease (Giddens and Sutton, 2017). Treatment is based upon interventions such as medication and surgical procedures by doctors and other qualified professionals. However, the recent growth in alternative medicine, such as homoeopathy, as another way to treat illness from a holistic perspective is becoming increasingly popular. People are now seeking other ways in which to treat sickness and disease. The practice of force-feeding, as seen in the case study, is a common and long-held tradition in some cultures to ensure that a child will remain healthy and well-fed. However, in Western culture, this would not be seen as the acceptable treatment of a child and would be viewed in terms of an act of cruelty.

It is easy to see from these three aspects of culture in relation to the case study that the concept is multifaceted and complex. The increasingly diverse nature of the population and various cultures (discussed in previous chapters) within modern Britain means that nurses are now, more than ever, likely to care for patients who have differing belief systems and concepts of health from their own. It is therefore important that an understanding of the components that lead to the development of cultural competence are a prerequisite to the delivery of appropriate, effective, and holistic nursing care (Henderson et al., 2018). It is impossible for you, as a student, to have knowledge of every culture or cultural identity. However, there is a need for nurses to be open and receptive to the development of their own individual cultural skill set (O'Hagan, 2001). In addition, as a nurse, you must also recognise and accept that your own beliefs, values, and culture can and will influence all your healthcare encounters. This calls for the skill of self-awareness, discussed in the previous chapter.

Complete Activity 4.1 to gain a better understanding of the concept of culture and its relevance in nursing, and to reflect on your own cultural background and identity following up from the introductory case study 'Nurse who force-fed her baby'.

## Activity 4.1 Reflection

In your own words, describe what you understand by the term 'culture'?

What is your cultural background or identity?

Make a list of some of the specific characteristics of your cultural background or identity.

Consider how the specific characteristics of your cultural background or identity influences your personal lifestyle, health, and relationship with others.

*Because this activity is based on your own thoughts, there is no model answer at the end of the chapter.*

In Activity 4.1 you would have identified that when we think about culture, we are referring to a shared way of life, belief systems, values, language, and ideas, as well as visibly expressed forms of customs, music, etiquette, and clothing of a group of people. This tells us that all human beings are cultural beings, and that culture will influence the lifestyle of an individual, their personal identity, and relationship with others (Papadopoulos, 2018) as you would have identified in your examples. These all have significant implications for healthcare and perceptions of health as evident from the case study.

In your role as a student nurse, it is worth remembering that even though culture can be a shared concept, it also tends to be unique to the individual (DeWilde and Burton, 2017). Just because two people share the same culture does not mean that they hold the same health beliefs and perform the same practices. The concept of culture can be misconstrued at times or even misused, as cultures are never homogenous and therefore it is important not to make generalisations about groups. Generalisations about groups are harmful as they lead to the development of stereotypes, misunderstanding of a culture, prejudice, and discrimination (Helman, 2007). In healthcare, culture may be overemphasised in how people present their symptoms as the symptoms or behaviour may be attributed to the person's culture. Pain as a symptom is a good example of how the generalisation of certain cultural groups can lead to poor care and discrimination in the healthcare setting and the management of pain. Black women, for example, are stereotyped as 'strong Black women', and feel that they are not seen, their concerns are not listened to or incorporated into their treatment decisions (NHS Race and Health Observatory, 2022). Such generalisation can lead to ineffective pain management for individuals in this group. One of the outcomes that you need to meet as part of your education and training is to provide and promote non-discriminatory, person-centred, and sensitive care at all times (NMC, 2018b), therefore it is important to not generalise. Finally, remember that you are bound by the Code (NMC, 2018a) and have a duty of care and candour to those in your care. You are required to take appropriate action should you witness any unlawful practices.

Having explored culture, this next section will explore the meaning of competence, competency, and cultural competency, in addition to some key supporting theories.

# Competence and cultural competency

## Competence

Becoming a registered nurse means that you are a professional, and therefore accountable for your practice; part of professionalism is the achievement of competence (NMC, 2017). The Code (NMC, 2018a) makes clear that nurses must practice effectively and preserve safety as a registered nurse, and performance that falls below this standard will be subject to scrutiny. You must also *recognise and work within the limits of your competence* (NMC, 2018a, p15). Essentially, nursing competence should be viewed as a holistic notion that encompasses not only the requisite knowledge and skills, but an appropriate attitude that conveys the unique art and skill of caring as a nurse. Competence is a generic quality and refers to an individual's capacity to perform job responsibilities, while competency is the actual performance or ability to do something in a specific situation (McConnell, 2001). Competent is defined as *having the necessary ability, knowledge or skill to do something successfully* (Lexico, 2019b).

It is important to define competence; that is, as a student nurse, successful achievement will allow you to register with the NMC. It also establishes the role of the nurse from a professional viewpoint (Fukada, 2018). Competence is gained through experience and learning, and it is described as a characteristic of behaviour (Fukada, 2018). As a student, you may already be familiar with a definition of competence or competency, as during your practice placements you are required to achieve a certain level of performance for successful progression. Throughout your training, you will complete mandatory training sessions, such as manual handling and lifting, and basic life support. These are necessary to ensure that when you attend practice placements, you are sufficiently prepared with the underpinning knowledge and understanding to perform specific tasks and skills. This does not mean that you are competent; you will need further practice in the clinical setting in order to develop.

A key issue with competence is that it can be dependent upon the particular situation or circumstance. Therefore, nurses are expected to use and adapt their underlying knowledge and skills to the environment in which they find themselves. In consideration of the above, the development and maintenance of competence and competency can be problematic if not practised on a regular basis so that you become familiar with the subject matter and skills involved (McConnell, 2001). That is why, in your role as a nurse, it is necessary, in line with the Code (NMC, 2018a), that you keep your knowledge and skills up to date. However, your attitude is just as important as your knowledge and skills, and during your clinical placements you will be aware that you are assessed in the three domains of knowledge, skill, and attitude. One of the findings from the Francis Report on the failings of the Mid-Staffordshire Trust was that some staff attitudes were described as 'leaving much to be desired' (Department of Health, 2013).

## Cultural competence

In discussing culture, it is evident that it impacts social behaviours and responses to health for both patients and healthcare professionals, and thus there is the need to be culturally competent because of the cultural diversity of the patients that access healthcare. There are various definitions of cultural competence, and it is universally acknowledged as an essential skill for healthcare professionals, as well as a prerequisite for positive health outcomes. The ongoing debate continues as to how to best define the concept of cultural competence, and within the literature there are different terminologies and definitions, of which the views of some theorists will be discussed.

The term 'cultural competence' was first coined by Madeleine Leininger in the 1960s as part of her theory of cultural care diversity and universality, and later used in published literature in the late 1980s (Shen, 2015). Madeleine Leininger (1925–2012) focused on transcultural nursing and cultural care (Leininger, 1978, 1988, 1995); she advocated the need for culturally competent nursing care due to the apparent lack of awareness of the need to recognise the importance of culture in care. Embedded in this was the need for nurses to be able to function effectively when caring for people from different cultures in her prediction of an increasingly multicultural world.

Irena Papadopoulos, Mary Tilki, and Gina Taylor produced together a model for the development of cultural competence in their work on defining cultural competence (Papadopoulos et al., 1998). Their definition sees cultural competence as providing effective healthcare to others while taking into consideration their cultural beliefs, behaviours, and needs. The term 'cultural competence' is seen as the end goal in the development of key skills such as cultural awareness, cultural sensitivity, and cultural knowledge, which are well-noted characteristics of the theory.

Another well-known leader in the field of cultural competence is Josepha Campinha-Bacote (2002), who described it as an ongoing process in which healthcare providers continually try to work in an effective manner within the cultural context of their clients. Simply put, it is the development of underpinning knowledge, skills, and attitudes in order to provide effective care to people from different cultural backgrounds.

Other definitions in the literature are by Cai (2016) in their concept analysis to give clarity to the term, identifying that cultural competence is a dynamic process with key defining characteristics for nurses to provide safe and quality healthcare that meets individual needs. The characteristics are cultural awareness, cultural sensitivity, cultural knowledge, and cultural skill. Also Henderson et al. (2018), in their concept analysis, provided another perspective on cultural competence in the context of healthcare in the community. The defining characteristics identified in their work were respecting and tailoring care, providing equitable and ethical care, and understanding. Henderson et al. (2018) put forward the argument for moral reasoning being key to cultural competence.

It is evident that cultural competence is a complex and multidimensional concept (Farber, 2019). It will continue to be discussed within nursing practice, as knowledge and skills are not static and will change in response to the needs of changing demographics within healthcare settings.

Your reading so far has introduced you to the meanings of competence and cultural competency, and how these underpin nursing practice. Activity 4.2 asks you to consider your own experience, preparation, and knowledge in the care of patients from different cultural groups.

## Activity 4.2   Reflection

For this activity, the aim is for you to focus on cultural competency for your field of practice.

Think about your last placement. How much information or preparation were you given by your practice assessor or supervisor about the different cultural groups/patients whom you might meet?

If you did not receive any information or preparation, what do you think you need to know and be prepared for when caring for diverse cultural groups/patients?

Choose a cultural group that you would like to find out more about. Take time out to research and make notes on the group you have chosen.

*There is a model answer at the end of the chapter.*

The consensus coming from the literature identifies some key characteristics that define cultural competence – cultural awareness, cultural sensitivity, cultural knowledge, and cultural skill. The next section will look at competence models and how they apply in the context of clinical practice. Read through the case scenarios and make some notes on the key cultural issues that stand out.

# Case scenarios

## Scenario 4.1

Imagine that you are admitting 55-year-old Sheila to the overnight stay surgical ward for a planned routine procedure. This is her first time being admitted to hospital, and Sheila did not want any treatment, but her symptoms of chronic tiredness and anaemia mean that she has been recommended for further examination. During the admission process, when you ask if she has any religious or spiritual beliefs, she tells you that she is a practising Jehovah's Witness. Sheila admits that she is nervous about the operation, and also that she was informed by the consultant that there was a possibility she might need a blood transfusion. As this is against her beliefs, she is adamant that she does not want this type of intervention. Sheila wants reassurance from you that she will not be given a blood transfusion.

## Scenario 4.2

Esme is a 68-year-old Jewish woman who has just been sectioned under the Mental Health Act 1983 as an inpatient on the mental health ward. Shanique, a first-year student nurse, is allocated to care for her with the supervision of her practice assessor. It is lunchtime, and Shanique brings Esme her kosher meal, and being helpful, proceeds to open the plastic covering. She is about to unwrap the cutlery when she notices that Esme has become very upset and tearful and refuses to eat the food. Esme will not explain why, and Shanique is confused and unsure of what to do. She leaves Esme to go to find her practice assessor for assistance.

## Scenario 4.3

Imagine you are a first-year student nurse on placement in the community and that you are spending some time with the health visitor, Nada, who is your practice supervisor. Bushra, a 25-year-old Muslim woman who has recently moved into the area, has brought her

2-year-old son, Jareem, for a developmental review and is terribly upset. Jareem is sitting on his mother's lap and is clingy towards her; he has a runny nose and a slight cough. Bushra is concerned about Jareem's recurrent cold and flu symptoms. She has seen the GP twice in the past six days for the symptoms and was advised by the GP that due to the frequency of his symptoms over the past six months he should be given the nasal flu vaccine; however, she has refused. Bushra becomes upset as she explains that her son is having frequent cold and flu symptoms and she does not know why. She also states that the GP keeps pushing her to agree to the flu vaccine being given to Jareem, but she is not happy about this. Bushra says that she has heard that the medicine contains gelatine and it is against her religious beliefs to allow him to have anything containing pork. Nada explains to Bushra that she has previously spoken to a number of Muslim parents about the flu vaccine and is happy to provide her with more information. In your student experience so far, you have not had much interaction with people from a Muslim background and are confused by Bushra's decision not to protect her child against recurrent cold and flu symptoms.

## Scenario 4.4

Vishal, age 35, has Down's Syndrome with challenging behaviours, and sensori-neural deafness for which he wears hearing aids. He lives at home with his parents, who manage his care with support from the Community Learning Disability Team. He has recently returned from a holiday visiting family in India with his parents, and has had severe diarrhoea since returning. You are a student nurse on placement with the Community Learning Disability Team, visiting Vishal for the first time since his return from holiday with your practice assessor (PA). On assessment by your PA, it is observed that he is lethargic, his mouth and skin are very dry, and he is also very quiet, which is unusual for him. His parents have been giving him herbal remedies to drink. It is evident that he is dehydrated, and your PA recommends that he needs to be taken to hospital. His parents refuse and your PA explains why he needs to go to hospital, but also wants to know why they are against this. Their concern is he will not be cared for properly as he has not had particularly good experiences, the hospital will not allow them to stay with him, and he may get COVID-19 or other infections worse than the diarrhoea by going into hospital.

# Cultural competence models

This section will look at cultural competence models. Before addressing cultural competence models, however, you need to understand the term 'models' in the context of nursing care. We will start with a discussion of the Roper–Logan–Tierney model of nursing, which is the most frequently used nursing model in the United Kingdom

(Roper et al., 2002). This model identifies 12 activities relevant to any individual's daily living and therefore can be applied across all fields of nursing. Within your field of practice, you will also use other nursing models relevant to the patient/client group and the setting where the care is being delivered. The purpose is to demonstrate the relevance of a nursing model before learning about models for cultural competence.

A key purpose of a nursing model is to collect information so that the nurse can perform a holistic patient assessment in a structured manner. You will then be able to develop an individualised plan that will facilitate and promote the continuity of care. By using a model, you can find out and review pertinent information that can be used to ascertain the patient's current and previous health status and identify nursing problems. From a professional perspective, according to Barrett et al. (2019), a model provides a picture of what nursing is and gives *direction to the nurse about patients and their needs, they define nursing roles* (p43).

The Roper–Logan–Tierney model (Roper et al., 2002) is founded upon the 12 activities of living (AL). All activities relate to an individual's day-to-day functioning and will be relevant to that. However, dependent upon the patient's circumstances, not all of the activities will be applicable at the time of the patient interaction.

These activities are:

- maintaining a safe environment
- communication
- breathing
- eating and drinking
- elimination
- personal cleansing and dressing
- controlling body temperature
- mobilising
- working and playing
- expressing sexuality
- sleeping
- dying

While these are applicable to every day across the lifespan, an individual's cultural needs may not be immediately obvious when using the model. It is therefore possible for you, as a student, to conduct an assessment using the AL model without it being alerted to any particular cultural values and preferences. This can happen between an inexperienced nurse and a patient who does not wish to divulge any cultural beliefs or values, particularly if they are not immediately apparent.

As a nurse, you will be aware that the first part of the nursing process is the patient assessment, which is discussed in more detail in Chapter 5. Assessment is key for you to collect valid and relevant information from your patient, and this can take time, dependent upon the type of admission. For example, in an emergency situation, there may not be much information that you can gather if the patient is unconscious. In that case, you would need to obtain information from other sources. Purnell (2016) stipulates that culturally congruent care will be achieved by gathering as much information as possible about the patient's culture during the assessment process. Culturally congruent care is that which *incorporates key values and beliefs of the client in a given situation* (Srivastava, 2003, p56). You will need to pay attention to the style of verbal and non-verbal communication employed by the patient, as well as your use of language that can be understood. This will help to build rapport and promote an environment in which the patient is comfortable enough to express their needs without fear of negative judgement or being misunderstood. The patient assessment will allow you to identify and prioritise the patient's problem. Remember that the patient assessment stage is an ongoing and continuous process, and not a one-off task, which is why Roper et al. (2002) prefer the term *assessing* rather than *assessment* (p124). Recommended resources for you to read more about this model are available at the end of the chapter.

# Cultural competence models and frameworks

We have looked at the purpose of a 'model' in the context of nursing to provide quality care. What was also highlighted with a model such as Roper et al. (2002) is that the impact of culture can easily be missed when assessing a patient. The need to provide quality care that is safe and takes into consideration cultural appropriateness is a key component of quality nursing care (Markey, 2021). This section will discuss three approaches to providing culturally competent care and inclusivity. The models discussed are the Papadopoulos model for culturally competent compassion (Papadopoulos, 2014), which has a focus on compassion in the quest to give culturally competent care, developing moral reasoning for culturally responsive care (Henderson et al., 2018; Markey, 2021), and the third approach will be cultural humility (Tervalon and Murray-García, 1998; Foronda et al., 2016; Lekas et al., 2020; Kelsall-Knight, 2022).

While you are reading this section, think about how skilled you consider yourself to be in each area and how you could demonstrate these skills in practical and theoretical terms.

## Papadopoulos's culturally competent compassion model (2014)

This model has a focus on compassion. The delivery of nursing care which shows compassion is of such significance that it is cited as one of the six Cs (care, compassion, competence, communication, courage, and commitment) (NHS England, 2015), which are benchmarks for the provision of nursing care that demonstrate the values of dignity and respect to patients.

The art of compassion has been defined by Perez-Bret et al. (2016) as:

> *the sensitivity shown in order to understand another person's suffering, combined with a willingness to help and to promote the well-being of that person, in order to find a solution to their situation.*

> (p605)

The authors also comment: *Compassionate care can be shown with words, but also by a silent, caring and respectful attitude* (p603).

Culturally competent compassion is defined by Papadopoulos and Pezella (2015) as:

> *the human quality of understanding the suffering of others and wanting to do something about it, using culturally appropriate and acceptable interventions, which take into consideration both the patients' and the carers' cultural backgrounds as well as the context in which care is given.*

> (p2)

The model of culturally competent compassion consists of four constructs from Papadopoulos' earlier work (Papadopoulos et al., 1998) with each construct linked to the need for compassion. This model focuses on developing the healthcare professional to be culturally competent and compassionate through:

*Cultural awareness and compassion:* This means having an awareness of our own cultural values and identity, as explored when discussing culture and how this may influence our behaviour. Consider Scenario 4.3 again and the actions of the GP towards Bushra to get the child vaccinated, did the GP consider exploring Bushra's beliefs and values?

*Cultural knowledge and compassion:* This demands a critical examination of how cultural beliefs inform our notion of compassion and a reflection of how our cultural similarities relate to and impact on compassion. Consider Scenario 4.4 and think about the family dynamics with Vishal and his parents, who are his main carers. Do you think that their wishes to not take him to hospital are acceptable and compassionate?

*Cultural sensitivity and compassion:* This is about developing culturally sensitive and compassionate therapeutic relationships. Communicating effectively and appropriately is key to this construct. In Scenario 4.2, do you think that Shanique recognised signs of emotional suffering in Esme or had the knowledge to do the right thing to meet her religious dietary requirements?

*Cultural competence and compassion:* This links to Papadopoulos' definition of culturally competent compassion and is the combination of the three previous constructs and the ability to apply all three constructs to ensure culturally appropriate interventions. Consider Scenario 4.3 again and the actions of Nada, the health visitor.

The key aspect of this model by Papadopoulos (2014) is the requirement for healthcare professionals to understand the concept and implications of cultural competence combined with the quality of compassion. The very nature of nursing means that without this, we cannot hope to practice effectively, nor see others and what they represent. A number of definitions have been provided above for the concept of compassion, and, as indicated by Papadopoulos (2014), it is a quality that is at the heart of clinical practice. Without compassion as a behavioural trait, care cannot be effective, nor humanely delivered, which without doubt is key in the delivery of culturally competent nursing care.

# Moral reasoning

Moral reasoning is reasoning based on evaluative judgements pertaining to others' welfare, rights, fairness, or justice based on moral principles (Dahl and Killen, 2018). In the context of ensuring culturally appropriate care, the need to articulate why it is not acceptable and unfair to disregard an individual's cultural needs is key. Henderson et al. (2018) developed a theoretical model of the concept of cultural competence in the context of providing culturally competent healthcare in the community. Their work identified that it was not sufficient to just have cultural knowledge and know about the patient's culture to be culturally competent, but to have a higher level of moral reasoning to sustain culturally competent practice. Markey (2021) highlights the need for nurses to examine cultural competence through a moral reasoning lens, as the model of morality can provide a framework exploring how moral motivation and behaviour occur, providing a way to critically examine the knowledge, skills, and attitudes to give culturally appropriate care.

Moral reasoning enables an individual to acknowledge when change is needed, which will occur when inconsistencies in principles or unequal treatment of others is noticed (Killen and Dahl, 2021). As a student this means applying moral reasoning in clinical decisions that you make by acknowledging when change is needed; by thinking about what is fair; by respecting and tailoring care to meet the needs of the patient; and by ensuring that the care provided is equitable ethical care. It will involve reflection on the care that you give when caring for culturally diverse patients, and examining your actions and omissions. This is a skill that will develop over time, and that you will learn from the various clinical experiences that you will encounter under supervision, including simulated practice learning.

# Cultural humility

Cultural competence is discussed widely in the literature and is also the approach that is advocated in healthcare. Cultural humility is a term first coined by Tervalon and Murray-García (1998) to move the shift from achieving cultural competence to achieving cultural humility in medical education. Cultural competence can contribute to the reproduction of stereotypes and an imbalance between patients and providers:

an argument put forward by Tervalon and Murray-García (1998) and which this chapter and previous chapters have touched on. Lekas et al. (2020) identify that cultures change because of interactions with others, institutions, media, technology, and the socio-economic determinants. Becoming 'competent' in any culture is therefore saying that the core sets of beliefs and values remain unchanged and are shared by all members of that group, which furthers arguments that this approach can possibly lead to stereotyping. Tervalon and Murray-García (1998, p123) define cultural humility as '*a lifelong commitment to self-evaluation and critique, to redressing power imbalances … and to developing mutually beneficial and non-paternalistic partnerships with communities on behalf of individuals and defined populations*'.

Applying cultural humility is about being aware of the imbalances in power that can occur within interactions in healthcare settings and being humble (Foronda et al., 2016). Chapters 1 and 2 have addressed key issues related to diversity in relation to health inequalities and cultural concepts of health. One of the key issues is the disparities in health and accessing healthcare by minoritised groups from the Black community and people of colour, the LGBTQIA+ community, and those living in rural areas or areas of poverty. The disparities as identified in the earlier chapters are largely influenced by such factors as structural racism and discrimination, implicit and explicit biases, unequal access to care, and unequal access to physical resources and environmental amenities. The presence of disparities contributes to the imbalances in power when patients from these groups access healthcare. These disparities can also be the reason why they may be reluctant to access healthcare or have certain treatments as a result of the biases they may experience, as reflected in the case scenarios.

As a student, you need to acknowledge that you have biases; the activities on reflecting on your own culture and how it influences you would have identified some of your biases. However, taking time to acknowledge and set aside the biases that will negatively impact patient care is key, as you have a duty of care to provide and promote non-discriminatory, person-centred, and sensitive care at all times (NMC, 2018b). Patient-centred care focuses on the needs of the patient, which will include their cultural needs, and therefore by nature it is anti-biased and anti-discriminatory.

In the context of nursing, the concept of cultural humility is about awareness of diversity and how an individual's culture can affect their health behaviours (Kelsall-Knight, 2022; Nolan et al., 2021). It is also about recognising the possible power imbalances in the nurse–patient relationship or a patient's relationships with other healthcare professionals that could affect patient outcomes (Corless et al., 2016). When applying cultural humility in practice you will need to demonstrate self-awareness, acknowledging that patients present with their lived experiences, thoughts, beliefs, and preferences for care as evident in the case scenarios. With regards to your practice, it must be anti-discriminatory: a requirement by the NMC (2018a, 2018b). In addition, you must be an active listener, acknowledging the concerns expressed by the patient. In summary, cultural humility is about openness, self-awareness, being humble, supportive: interactions, self-reflection, critique, and the consequence of all these attributes lead to mutual empowerment, respect, partnership, optimal care, and lifelong learning (Nolan et al., 2021). Activity 4.3 now explores how you can apply these to your practice.

## Activity 4.3   Reflection

Reflecting on your field of practice, revisit the case scenarios again and what you identified as the key cultural issues. Now think of the different approaches such as cultural humility and moral reasoning and how you can apply these in practice to promote culturally appropriate care.

*There are model answers on this activity and the case scenarios at the end of the chapter.*

This section has provided you with an understanding of the underpinning theory and its applications. There are other cultural competence models contained in nursing literature that you can research in your own time, to widen your knowledge base in this subject area. By using the models and frameworks discussed, the nurse can engage in a meaningful way with the patient, which will promote understanding and collaboration in order to positively address healthcare needs.

## Chapter summary

Cultural competence does not necessarily mean that the healthcare professional is an expert in all aspects of this field. However, the recognition that culture is a fundamental part of the nursing role and of the patients we meet is a well-intentioned starting point.

Inevitably, during your practice, you will come across individuals from different cultures with values and beliefs that are unlike your own. Cultural skill awareness and the ongoing pursuit of cultural competence is a requirement for all healthcare professionals, in order to address the needs of patients from different backgrounds. Competence needs to be demonstrated in meaningful ways through education and exposure to practice so that skills can be improved. Communication and a desire to deliver quality care that is respectful and demonstrates dignity to those with different cultural needs and beliefs should be a common goal for all those involved in the delivery of nursing care. As a nurse, reflect on your clinical skill, knowledge, and practice in terms of how you relate to and care for patients in a culturally appropriate manner. Take the opportunity to discuss cultural care with your practice assessor and others in the clinical environment. It is to our detriment, in today's society, if we fail to do so.

# Activities: brief outline answers

## Activity 4.2　Reflection (p75)

It is good practice to make a conscious effort in each clinical placement you attend to ask questions about the different cultures of patients admitted to the ward and consider setting one of your learning objectives for placement to address the development of cultural competency. The placement area should have guidelines that relate specifically to the most common cultural groups that you will encounter, so make sure that you read them. Actions that you can apply when you initially care for a patient from a different culture and what questions you can ask to deliver culturally appropriate care could include:

- Reading the patient's medical and nursing notes and familiarise yourself with relevant information, such as language spoken, reason for admission, diagnosis, and current health status.
- Before approaching the patient (you may be in the company of your practice assessor), ensure that you are clear as to what you are going to be doing with/to the patient (i.e. that you are working within your limitations).
- Introduce yourself and ask if they have a preferred name/title that they would like to be known as.
- Do not be afraid to ask the patient questions in an appropriate manner about their cultural background; most patients will not mind as long as you explain your reason for doing so.
- If the situation allows, find out as much information as you can about the patient's preferences, values, beliefs, and traditions, particularly if they may have implications on the hospital stay. Do not forget to include significant others and family members.
- Document the information you obtain in the patient's notes and inform your practice assessor.
- Think about any possible challenges in the ward environment that may hinder the provision of cultural care to your patient.
- Discuss the encounter with your practice assessor or supervisor and reflect on the interaction.

## Activity 4.3　Reflection (p83)

### Scenario 4.1

The key issue for Sheila is her religion and how this has an influence on the types of healthcare interventions she can have, and this is causing her some level of anxiety as she does not want to have any treatment. The assessment will need to factor in her religious beliefs and address these with sensitivity and respect, as it impacts what type of treatment she can have. Her anxieties will need to be communicated to the consultant. As the nurse, you will need self-awareness to respond to her needs, as the model requires you to understand how the patient views and explains the problem. It is also key to ensure that Sheila feels culturally safe in order to reduce her anxiety, which is part of maintaining a safe environment. This is concerned with the internal and external environment and harm can come from many sources. What you do need to be aware of, appreciate and respect are the beliefs of Jehovah's Witnesses not to accept blood transfusions (Jehovah's Witnesses, 2018). Chapter 6 addresses in more depth religion, spirituality, and faith.

### Scenario 4.2

The key issue for Esme again relates to religion, but in this case her dietary needs. Esme is Jewish. There was a lack of understanding of her needs by Shanique. Adequate nutritional intake is necessary for patient recovery and well-being and is part of the activity of living, eating, and drinking. Shanique as a first-year student has recognised this and is being helpful by trying to ensure that Esme can eat. In some cultural groups, there are strict rules to be followed concerning dietary habits and religion is usually the most common reason for food restrictions. Jewish traditions concerning dietary habits are that all meals must be prepared and served by the observance of *kashrut,* which are kosher laws (Spritzer, 2003). In the hospital setting, the hospital kosher meals service will undertake this responsibility. All food must be served in specially sealed containers with disposable cutlery and given to the patient without breaking the seal or disturbing the cutlery. Esme is likely to be experiencing a range of emotions, such as feeling shocked and upset that her religious beliefs have not been sufficiently considered. For Esme to feel culturally safe, any care interventions should aim at being orientated to her values and beliefs, showing sensitivity. As a student nurse caring for these individuals, you must appreciate the impact of religious beliefs and their importance in relation to care delivery (Mendes, 2015). If, as a student, you are unsure about dietary habits, the easiest way to find out is to ask the patient, as they are usually more than willing to explain their specific requirements. As you can now understand, due to a lack of knowledge, the result of inadequate nutritional intake will have repercussions on health and the delivery of individualised patient care. This calls for sensitivity and underscores the need to ensure a holistic cultural patient assessment in which relevant needs are addressed.

## Scenario 4.3

The key issue in this scenario for Bushra is about vaccine hesitancy and the approach by the GP, her faith as a Muslim, and the health of Jareem. Application of the ACCESS model in this case scenario can help respond to the diverse needs of Bushra. Nada will need to be sensitive when discussing the issue of vaccination administration, given that it does contain porcine (a derivative of pork), which is strictly prohibited in Muslim culture. Nada will need to allow Bushra the time to speak about her concerns, paying attention to both verbal as well as non-verbal cues. It is important to find out specifically what Bushra wants to know and what she wants to achieve at the end of the discussion. This can help to guide the amount and type of information provided. Nada will need to explain fully to her the ingredients of the nasal flu vaccine and, if appropriate, suggest the possibility of an alternative injection that does not contain any porcine (PHE, 2014). Consideration needs to be made in terms of the benefits of vaccination. It is also important to consider any past medical history that Jareem might have. Advice should be given to Bushra on aspects of daily living that might be making Jareem more susceptible to colds and flu, such as diet and home environment. It is important that Bushra's wishes are respected and that she does not feel that she is being forced into making decisions with which she is not happy. More information can be provided to Bushra to aid her understanding so that she can make a fully informed decision that does not go against her beliefs. At the end of the discussion, Nada should ask Bushra to recall what she has been told to ensure clarity and understanding. However, it is important to ascertain Bushra's level of literacy as this will impact on the processing of information she is given. Nada should have a discussion with the GP to advise them of the outcome of the consultation and to explain cultural variations, such as Bushra's lack of engagement, if they are unaware of these.

## Scenario 4.4

Vishal is unwell and needs to be in hospital as he is dehydrated. However, his parents are reluctant for him to be taken to hospital due to previous experiences. They have been managing him at home with herbal remedies. In this scenario, what is in the best interest of Vishal, who has Down's Syndrome, while being culturally sensitive to his parents' approach to his needs as his main carers, is important, and has to be managed with sensitivity and respect. Further assessment of health beliefs and practices will be relevant, and even if Vishal is lethargic, he should still be part of the assessment and discussions. His parents are also thinking of his best interest, and as a family they need to have a feeling of cultural safety in the sense of Vishal's disabilities, age, abilities, and ethnicity. It is evident that his parents find the hospital alienating and therefore it can be described as culturally unsafe for them and this needs to be addressed to prevent further deterioration in Vishal's health. Assessment of the activities of living will identify his physical health needs, informing the decision for Vishal to be taken to hospital. The assessment can be enhanced to address the understanding of the parents through cultural negotiation and compromise, in order to come to an agreement concerning what is in the best interests of Vishal. There is already a therapeutic relationship as the family have been supported by the Community Learning Disability Team. This scenario also highlights the balance of power, as discussed in the section on cultural humility.

# Further reading

**Barrett, D, Wilson, B, and Woollands, A** (2019) *Care Planning: A Guide for Nurses* (3rd edn). London: Routledge.

Chapter 3 gives the reader an underpinning theory in relation to the activities of the living model.

**Papadopuolos, I** (2018) *Culturally Competent Compassion: A Guide for Healthcare Students and Practitioners.* London: Routledge.

# Useful websites

Cultural Competence: e-Learning for Healthcare:

**www.e-lfh.org.uk/programmes/cultural-competence/**

This is an e-learning tool developed by Health Education England in partnership with the Royal College of Midwives to assist healthcare professionals in developing their knowledge and skills in aspects of culture and health. You will have to register on the site unless you already have an account with e-Learning for Healthcare.

**Papadopoulos, I** (2014) *The Papadopoulos Model for Developing Culturally Competent Compassion in Healthcare Professionals.*

**www.youtube.com/watch?v=zjKzO94TevA** (accessed 16 November 2022).

This is a short YouTube video that provides an overview of the components of the model.

# Chapter 5

# Assessing the needs of diverse patients

*Mariama Seray-Wurie and Beverley Brathwaite*

## NMC Future Nurse: Standards of Proficiency for Registered Nurses

This chapter will address the following platforms and proficiencies:

**Platform 1: Being an accountable professional**

1.4 demonstrate an understanding of, and the ability to challenge, discriminatory behaviour.

1.9 understand the need to base all decisions regarding care and interventions on people's needs and preferences, recognising and addressing any personal and external factors that may unduly influence your decisions.

1.14 provide and promote non-discriminatory, person-centred and sensitive care at all times, reflecting on people's values and beliefs, diverse backgrounds, cultural characteristics, language requirements, needs and preferences, taking account of any need for adjustments.

**Platform 2: Promoting health and preventing ill health**

2.2 demonstrate knowledge of epidemiology, demography, genomics, and the wider determinants of health, illness, and well-being and apply this to an understanding of global patterns of health and well-being outcomes.

2.3 understand the factors that may lead to inequalities in health outcomes.

2.10 provide information in accessible ways to help people understand and make decisions about their health, life choices, illness, and care.

**Platform 3: Assessing needs and planning care**

3.4 understand and apply a person-centred approach to nursing care, demonstrating shared assessment, planning, decision-making, and goal setting when working with people, their families, communities, and populations of all ages.

3.5 demonstrate the ability to accurately process all information gathered during the assessment process to identify needs for individualised nursing care and develop person-centred evidence-based plans for nursing interventions with agreed goals.

*(Continued)*

(Continued)

### Platform 4: Providing and evaluating care

4.1　demonstrate and apply an understanding of what is important to people and how to use this knowledge to ensure their needs for safety, dignity, privacy, comfort, and sleep can be met, acting as a role model for others in providing evidence-based person-centred care.

4.2　work in partnership with people to encourage shared decision-making in order to support individuals, their families, and carers to manage their own care when appropriate.

### Platform 7: Coordinating care

7.1　understand and apply the principles of partnership, collaboration and inter-agency working across all relevant sectors.

## Chapter aims

After reading this chapter, you will be able to:

- examine the impact of diverse cultural influences affecting health beliefs and perceptions of illness on those in your care;
- reflect on your own beliefs about health and illness, diversity and culture, and how this may influence your assessment and perception of an individual in your care; and
- describe key techniques that can be utilised when assessing an individual in your care to ensure recognition of diversity and avoidance of assumptions.

# Introduction

## Scenario 5.1

Martha, a 68-year-old trans woman of colour presented to the emergency department with chest pain. Following assessment and investigation, it is confirmed that Martha has had a myocardial infarction and is admitted to the coronary care unit. Martha was allocated to a side room. During her time as an inpatient her physical appearance was disconcerting to some staff. Martha was aware of the glares and whispers from certain nursing staff, who were visibly uncomfortable with their interactions with her, especially when communicating, as they would have difficulty maintaining eye contact and were unsure about what was or was not appropriate during her care as she had a limited nursing assessment completed due to this uncomfortableness. Martha raised her concerns about how she was being treated and made to feel by certain staff with the ward manager but did not want to make an official complaint. As a result of this feedback, the ward manager decided to address this with the ward staff and students during the handover. The manager started the conversation by quoting:

> *The NHS provides a comprehensive service, available to all irrespective of gender, race, disability, age, sexual orientation, religion, belief, gender reassignment, pregnancy and maternity or marital or civil partnership status. The service is designed to improve, prevent, diagnose and treat both physical and mental health problems with equal regard. It has a duty to each and every individual that it serves and must respect their human rights. At the same time, it has a wider social duty to promote equality through the services it provides and to pay particular attention to groups or sections of society where improvements in health and life expectancy are not keeping pace with the rest of the population.*
>
> (United Kingdom Government, 2021)

Staff were then asked if they thought this was happening on the ward and to give examples of this.

The above scenario and quote used highlights the first principle stated in the NHS Constitution outlining the need to provide a service to all, and within this statement there is an acknowledgement of diversity.

Part of the acknowledgement of diversity within healthcare is about appreciating how an individual perceives health and illness and influencing factors on these phenomena. Nursing has a pivotal role in the delivery of care within the NHS and users of the service will at some point need to have an assessment undertaken by a nurse. Your own views of diversity, health, and illness, and your culture will influence to some extent how you deliver care, as nurses are from diverse backgrounds. Assessment and care planning is one of the principles in the NMC Standards of Proficiency for Registered Nurses (NMC, 2018a), and in line with the Code (NMC, 2018b) it is a requirement to treat people as individuals, avoid making assumptions, recognising diversity and individual choice.

This chapter will allow you to explore your own perceptions of health and illness, diversity, and culture, as your personal understanding of these issues is pivotal in the assessment and planning of care to ensure that your own beliefs do not influence care in an inappropriate way. A significant part of the nurse's role involves working with diverse groups, individuals, and families in a variety of healthcare settings. There are many challenges when working with a diverse patient group with different cultures, as the individual will have their own health belief systems that may be influenced by their culture, religion, age, gender, or sexuality.

This chapter will also examine how personal beliefs from the patient perspective influence health and illness, especially from disadvantaged minority groups, and how these may not always correspond with Western medicine and the biomedical approach to care. It will address concepts around cultural competency, and the final part of the chapter will focus on exploring ways to ensure equality and inclusivity when assessing and planning care with diverse patient groups.

# Why can assessment be complex when managing diverse and culturally different patients?

Assessment in the context of healthcare is a complex process that is completed by a registered healthcare professional, and, as a student, you will be supervised in carrying out this activity. It is not just a one-off process as it will be an activity that continues throughout the relationship between you, as a nurse, with the patient/service user and their family where applicable. It is the first step that is undertaken in order to plan care, and as such the assessment which should identify the individual's health needs, but also give insight into their beliefs and perception of their health and illness. To undertake this activity, as a nurse, you have to be able to utilise good communication skills such as good questioning techniques and listening skills, be observant of responses and body language, and have an open mind and not be judgemental. It is vital that all aspects of the individual's health and illness are explored to formulate a plan of care that will address the needs of the individual and their family where applicable. The process can be described as doing detective work, and as such, even though you may rely on scientific knowledge of the health problem and your own instinctive beliefs, using these solely would result in key problems not being identified correctly or being missed. An assessment in all cases needs to be holistic, addressing physical, psychological, and sociological aspects of care and how health has been affected as a result of the illness. Building a therapeutic relationship between the nurse and patient will ensure that, as a nurse, you explore the individual's perception of how they feel about their health/illness and influencing factors. Individuals and families will conceptualise illness and how it is treated in different ways; this may not be congruent with your expectations, which may possibly lead to you, as a nurse, being prejudiced or judgemental by not recognising or understanding these differing influences. It is therefore relevant for you, as a student, to reflect on some of your own beliefs, values, and culture to explore how this could possibly influence negatively or even positively how you assess individuals from diverse backgrounds. To do this, you will need to address reflective learning as in Activity 5.1.

## Activity 5.1   Teamworking

Looking at Scenario 5.1 how do you think the issue of both communication and teamwork could be resolved to improve the care that Martha received?

*There is an outline answer at the end of the chapter.*

Now that you have thought about your cultural awareness, let us look at how it impacts nursing assessment and care delivery. This will be followed by some scenarios to get you to link in 'real-life' situations.

# Cultural awareness

Just learning about other cultures does not always equate to having cultural awareness as a nurse. To develop cultural awareness, self-examination and understanding of one's own cultural beliefs and values related to healthcare and the profession is key.

An individual may respond to illness the way they do because of their cultural background or in response to how they may have been treated in the past because of their cultural diversity. This may have occurred from a nurse or any other healthcare professional due to a lack of awareness of cultural practices other than their own, or a lack of appreciation of the diversity of individuals and making assumptions. It is an expectation that nurses are able to assess and plan care that is clinically safe and culturally sensitive. However, when undertaking an activity such as assessment, the outcome may be an incorrect interpretation of the individual's needs or becoming frustrated with the individual or their family if there is a lack of cultural sensitivity or appreciation of diversity. This goes against Platform 1, 'Being an accountable professional', which states that registered nurses act in the best interests of people, putting them first and providing nursing care that is person-centred, safe, and compassionate (NMC, 2018a).

The beliefs of the individual play a significant role when assessing and planning care to foster partnership with the individual and their family where relevant. The consensus within nursing from the Royal College of Nurses (RCN) about those who enter the profession is the desire to help people (RCN, 2019). From Activity 5.1, you should have recognised that even though, as a student nurse, you are compassionate and care for your patients with good intentions, your personal background, culture, education, race, gender, sexual orientation, age, or religion have influenced, and always will influence, to some extent, how you deliver nursing care. You may at this stage, at the start of your career as a student, find these thoughts challenging as you may feel that you are not providing the best care due to your own beliefs. Almaturi and Rodney (2013) identified that when viewing and interpreting the world, people will tend to use their own cultural lens to evaluate others' behaviours, which may or may not lead to tension and conflict. However, it is not always a negative attribute if you are aware of how your beliefs influence the nursing care you give and the potential of how it may affect the way you see the patient as an individual. If applying some of the defining attributes of being culturally competent as identified by Henderson et al. (2018), such as respecting and tailoring care aligned with the patient's values, needs, practices, and expectations; and delivering equitable and ethical care to the health condition, both mental as well as physical, the care they require should not be impacted on negatively.

## Scenario 5.2

You are on placement with the health visitor (HV) on a visit to the Bada family, who have settled in the UK as refugees. Their eldest child, Yasmin, age 5, has severe physical and developmental delays as a result of a lack of oxygen at birth. The HV would like, with the consent of the parents, to refer the child for an intensive physiotherapy and occupational health programme that would help her to become more independent. The parents, Joseph and Mariam, are declining to give consent as they state it is their duty to care for Yasmin, as they believe that Yasmin's condition is punishment for conceiving her before they were married, and as such it is their burden to care for her. The HV is upset with the parents and feels that Jacob and Mariam are not acting in the best interest of Yasmin.

## Scenario 5.3

Ms Tran arrives at the urgent care centre with her 12-year-old son, Giang. She is Vietnamese and does not speak English, but her son Giang does, and he is interpreting for his mother. Ms Tran has severe abdominal pain and vaginal bleeding. She is clutching her lower abdomen and appears visibly distressed, as does Giang, who states he is scared that something will happen to his mother. The nurse who is assigned to the case informs Giang that they are going to get an interpreter so that they can assess Ms Tran, and in the meantime, he can go to the play area and wait. Ms Tan and Giang both become very upset as they do not want to be separated.

## Scenario 5.4

Errol, age 58, has a long history of mental health problems and type 2 diabetes. He is known to the community mental health services as he is on medication that is supervised by them, as he is divorced and lives alone in a Council flat. He has lost sensation in his lower limbs and has sustained a burn injury to the sole of his left foot from a hot water bottle. He has not had the wound assessed by a health professional as he dressed it himself. The community mental health services, on their visit, decide to quickly assess the wound, and on taking off the bandage discover a picture of St Francis of Assisi covered in plastic between the layers of the bandage. Errol describes the picture as a relic that can prevent or positively influence life's problems, and that St Francis is known for healing animals and people; therefore, having the picture in the dressing will help the wound to heal.

## Scenario 5.5

Krishnan, age 37, has recently been diagnosed with chronic renal failure. He has started peritoneal dialysis, and as part of his management, maintaining adequate protein intake is an essential part of his ongoing treatment, of which animal protein is the recommended source. Krishnan is Hindu by religion and has eaten chicken and eggs all his life. However, since the diagnosis, he has decided to become a vegetarian as he wants to become a good Hindu so that God will help him with his ordeal. He states that not eating meat is a more devout way of life and one he wishes to follow.

## Scenario 5.6

Jonathan, age 32, has autistic spectrum disorder (ASD) and is partially sighted. He was admitted to the surgical ward following emergency surgery for a bowel obstruction. He has received a visit from his support worker from the learning disabilities team that supports him in the community, as he lives in sheltered housing. The support worker notices that Jonathan appears withdrawn and uncommunicative. He has been on the ward for two days and the staff have attended to his medical and physical needs, but left him alone most of the time.

Looking at these scenarios, you should now start to have an awareness of the complexities involved when undertaking a patient assessment with diverse patient groups and their beliefs. From Activity 5.1, you should be able to conclude that the individuals and their families have a unique identity, influenced by how they see themselves with regard to personal background, culture, education, race, gender, sexual orientation, disability, age, or religion. Therefore, as a nurse, focusing on only one aspect of their identity is counterproductive when undertaking assessment and planning of care, as there is the potential for you to stereotype. Although stereotypes can be positive as well as negative, from the negative perspective, if you have a stereotypical view of the individual in your care, it can hinder communication (Jandt and Jandt, 2018) and create bias, which in turn will cause barriers in the working relationship with your patient. When there are barriers, the outcome will be a plan of care that does not meet the needs of the individual, and possibly care that is substandard as a result of the nurse and other health professionals not factoring in the wider cultural and diverse influences (Papadopoulos, 2006). In addition to the NMC Standards and the NMC Code, which clearly state the need to recognise and respect difference, as a student, you must also be aware of relevant legislation that is key with regard to the commitment to promote equality and stop unlawful racial discrimination (see Chapter 2 on the Equality Act, 2010). As a nurse, it is therefore vital to be aware of individual differences (Griffith, 2009). It can be argued that it is not possible for the nurse to understand and be competent in the assessment and planning of care for every diverse group, as the UK is very culturally, ethnically, and linguistically diverse, with a significant LGBTQIA+ population and a growing elderly population, and with improvements in healthcare provision, people with disabilities and long-term conditions are living longer. However, this should not deter you, as identified by O'Hagan (2001), who advocates that *how you approach* someone who is from a different culture is more important than being highly knowledgeable about the differences.

## Activity 5.2    Critical Thinking

How would you respond to the scenarios described above and why?

*This is an activity to be done from your perspective, based on your personal values and beliefs; therefore, there is no outline answer at the end of the chapter. However, there are some valuable points to consider, outlined at the end of the chapter.*

Having got some clarity on the impact of personal beliefs and the need to appreciate difference, we can now consider the patient and family perspective in Activity 5.3.

## Activity 5.3    Critical thinking

Now look again at the five previous scenarios. What factors do you think influence perceptions of illness from the patient and family perspective, and what is the relevance of this when assessing an individual?

Thinking about the patient's perspective can only help with being able to make the right clinical decisions with and for the patient.

*An outline of what you might find is given at the end of the chapter.*

# Relevance of patients' beliefs to the assessment process

When assessing a patient, for this to be truly holistic, understanding cultural beliefs and having an appreciation of differences must be a fundamental part of the assessment process and planning of care, as does an appreciation of the diversity of the patient. This will ensure that the care for the patient is culturally appropriate. Evidence in the literature (Bjarnason et al., 2009; Meddings and Hiath-Cooper, 2008) shows that in situations when care is not culturally appropriate, this leads to an undesirable course of events, from miscommunication to life-threatening incidents.

Understanding the health beliefs of the individual is key when assessing the patient, as perception of illness and the cause varies by culture and individual preferences, which will influence how you assess and deliver care as a nurse. For care to be inclusive of culture and diversity, it must combine the beliefs, values, and attitudes of the patient and their family where relevant with the values that are subscribed to within healthcare provision, which tends to be mainly based on Western values and the biomedical model of care. Issues of conflict may arise when a healthcare professional disregards or fails to appreciate other influences outside of the biomedical model and Western practices.

Let us look again at the five scenarios above (Scenarios 5.2–5.6). You were asked to think of how the nurses responded, which should have again highlighted how personal beliefs and values would have influenced the reaction. You were also asked to think about the scenarios from the patient perspective; Activity 5.2 outlines some of the cultural factors from a patient perspective. The scenarios touch lightly on some factors that influence beliefs in health and illness within diverse patient groups. Individuals will have different views about the origin, causes, and best way to treat illness, and, as a nurse, this must be recognised when undertaking patient assessment and applied to all diverse groups. Even a child or young person has their beliefs about illness, and this must be respected (UN Convention, 1990). Culture is a clear factor that influences belief; however, it is also key to recognise that even though you may have individuals from the same background, this does not necessarily mean they believe in the same cultural practices, and therefore you should not assume this. Religion, which will be discussed in Chapter 6, influences beliefs regarding health and illness, and again the same principle applies with regard to making assumptions as religion in itself has diverse practices. Going back to Scenarios 5.2 and 5.4, it is evident that the beliefs held in the scenarios do not match up with what you perceive as a duty of care, as a nurse, but also a lack of awareness or understanding of an individual's customs. Getting to know your patient and the perceptions of their illness is a generic principle that is applied in all aspects of nursing care, and where there are beliefs that may not be congruent with the evidence that clinical practice is based on, it is about working in partnership with the individual to see how their needs can be best met. This is where your listening and observational skills are important when you are undertaking assessment. In addition to the issues of culture and religion, other factors, such as gender, education, socio-economic background, career, and family traditions, will influence an individual's perception of health and illness (Griffith, 2009). From the assessment and when planning the care, it is about having a balance. This means utilising both the patient's influences and the scientific evidence. It may be that you are of the opinion that the biomedical approach to illness is best, and indeed this may be a fact; however, if the patient and their family do not see it this way, then to address this complexity an egalitarian or open approach needs to be evident. In the past and with biomedical models, a paternalistic approach was taken with patients; however, as the population has grown and become more diverse, other factors that influence health and illness have become very evident, and legislation such as the Equality Act 2010 means that within healthcare settings, care has to be delivered that recognises and supports the equality of all people, taking on board their needs by working in partnership with the patient and their family.

# How to ensure equality and inclusivity when assessing and planning care for diverse patient groups

To provide and promote non-discriminatory, person-centred, and sensitive care at all times as outlined by the NMC (2018a), a nurse should be culturally aware, culturally knowledgeable, and culturally sensitive in their practice. Recognising the diverse nature of the users of the health service is the first step. Then understanding their needs should follow to develop the relationship value, and this understanding of needs must be taken into consideration for care to be personalised. However, given the wide range of diverse groups of patients, it is not possible to have an understanding of every diverse group and their cultural practices; therefore, it should be the approach to diversity and cultural differences that is key. When undertaking patient assessment, the outcome is to understand what the patient's needs are. These needs are unique to the patient and will include clinical symptoms that need medical/nursing attention and issues specific to the individual that can affect their care. When undertaking patient assessment, it is important for you to be prepared to address not just the clinical symptoms, but also the spectrum of demographics and personal characteristics that will influence individual beliefs and responses to health and illness. In Activity 5.2, you should have identified cultural data in the scenarios that are part of the spectrum of demographics and personal characteristics.

As part of the assessment process in nursing, you will use various assessment tools to help gather clinical data about the patient that is structured and ensures an effective assessment.

## Activity 5.4   Reflection

Think of the scenarios that have been discussed. Reflecting on clinical practice and the nursing models and assessment tools that are used as part of the data-gathering process and care planning, do you think the models and tools you are familiar with capture the diverse needs of the patient groups to ensure that the outcome of the assessment and care planned is inclusive?

*As this is an activity for you to reflect on what you have observed in practice and your own personal thoughts, there is no model answer at the end of the chapter.*

Roper et al.'s (2002) *model of living* and the *12 activities of living* is a common model utilised in nursing practice. In addition to this model there are others that could be utilised within the scenarios as part of the assessment, such as the Malnutrition Universal Screening Tool (MUST), SSKIN bundle (Surface, Skin inspection, Keep moving, Incontinence, Nutrition), Wound assessment tools, National Early Warning Scores (NEWS), Paediatric Early Warning Score (PEWS), Mini-Mental State Examination (MMSE), 4AT Rapid Clinical Test for Delirium, Pain assessment tools, the Distress and Discomfort Assessment Tool (DisDAT), and Traffic Light Assessment. You may be questioning if the patient understands the purpose of these tools and if the tools are inclusive. Wilson et al. (2018) identify some of the limitations of using assessment tools in nursing, such as over-reliance on the tool, which can lead to missing other issues going on with the patient, and in the context of diversity, assessment tools may not be culturally sensitive and could again miss out on significant aspects of the patient's needs. Lifestyle, health beliefs, and health practices should be captured in a comprehensive holistic assessment and must involve the patient and family or carer where relevant.

Outlined are some examples of the challenges that you may come across within the assessment process and the reliance on tools that may not be culturally sensitive or promote inclusivity.

## Assessment of patients with dark-pigmented skin

*Skin colour matters in health care. Clinicians make decisions based on colour assessments multiple times each day as they gauge tissue perfusion and assess for jaundice, pallor, cyanosis, and the blanch response.*

(Everett et al., 2012, p496)

This statement identifies the growing field of research on the important practicalities of understanding that not all skin pigmentation is the same, and what is being done to address this. The focus should be on the physiology of the skin, and not the socially constructed attributes connected to skin colour, such as race, ethnicity, culture, religion, and language, although research on pressure ulcer assessment finds that making this distinction can be difficult in healthcare, as in society. Oozageer Gunowa et al. (2018) found that detecting pressure damage in people with darker skin tones is mainly focused on ethnicity and race rather than variations in skin pigmentation. The patient's skin tone should be the focus of the assessment allowing for individualised care (Oozageer Gunowa et al., 2018). What happens when we do not assess patients with dark-pigmented skin adequately for pressure damage is that erythema and category 1 pressure ulcers are at higher risk of pressure ulcer development, and they are more likely to go undetected and deteriorate (Baker, 2016; Sullivan, 2014).

*Rather than exercising 'color blindness' when assessing and treating patients, practitioners should exercise 'color awareness' by adjusting interventions and assessment techniques using the patients' physiological characteristics rather than depending on racial or ethnic categorization to guide care (Sommers, 2011).*

(Everett et al., 2012, p507)

This is an essential point that you need to carry with you when assessing all patients, but particularly those with darker skin tones, when carrying out a visual assessment, whether it be cyanosis or eczema in children (Myers, 2015).

It is vital to develop your knowledge on how to assess in other ways, taking into consideration skin pigmentation. In the 'Further reading' section below, we direct you to resources that will be useful to you in learning what can be done and practising this in your clinical placements.

## Assessment and issues related to gender

Within nursing, you will encounter people, including children, who identify themselves differently from the sex they were assigned at birth. Gender diversity is not a new phenomenon (Richards and Barret, 2020a). Gender identity is a key part of the people we care for. It will not be uncommon as a student to be involved in the assessment and care of a gender-diverse or trans person and to want to do 'the right thing' but unsure what this may be as this is not something that stands out in the assessment models and tools. A trans person using the NHS is more than often let down by the service as they encounter significant problems due to attitudes from some clinicians, lack of knowledge, and in some instances prejudice (Assessment, 2022; House of Commons Women and Equalities Committee, 2016). Doing the 'right thing' will involve creating a safe environment for the patient by being polite, not overthinking or fretting, and a key point on what you can do when assessing to promote inclusivity with all patients would include asking the patient what their preferred terms are and to use those. You should also bear in mind that trans people who have been in contact with mental health services may be exhausted by the constant assessment or exploration of their gender, therefore minimise questioning related to this and focus on the current problem they have presented with and not the 'trans' aspect (Richards and Barrett, 2020b). Considering the scenario at the start of the chapter about Martha, how do you think the assessment and care of Martha could have been more person-centred and culturally appropriate?

## Assessment and issues related to ageism

As stated by the World Health Organisation (WHO), ageism arises when age is used to categorise and divide people in ways that lead to harm, disadvantage, and injustice (WHO, 2021). It can affect any age group, therefore an appreciation of the impact of ageism on health is relevant for your practice as a nurse, even though most of the existing evidence in the literature focuses on the impact on older adults. The impact of ageism across the life span is said to stem from the perception that an individual may be too old or too young to be or to do something (Officer and de la Fuente-Núñez, 2018). Ageism, unlike other forms of discrimination such as sexism and racism, is socially acceptable as it is mainly implicit and subconscious in nature. Culturally, stereotypes of ageing focus on negative aspects. For example, typecasting ageing as a decline in physical and mental capacity, becoming dependent (Officer and de la Fuente-Núñez, 2018), or in the case of younger adults and children, their voices are often denied or dismissed (WHO, 2021). Another example of typecasting within different cultures is seeing the older person as a wise person to be valued. The impact on health from these stereotypes can be wide-ranging and this may even be some of your own cultural stereotypes of ageing; thus it can have an impact on how you undertake an assessment. A key area that you need to be aware of in your practice is that patterns of migration mean the ageing population includes a growing number of older people from a wide range of Minority Ethnic groups, which requires you to be appreciative of their different cultural and religious beliefs when assessing this group. For example, if the older person is seen as a wise individual the family will have different views and expectations about their care. Acknowledge their life experiences and how these may have impacted their health when gathering health information, and incorporate this information into the planning of the care as the assessment tools may not capture this information.

## Assessment and issues related to refugees and people seeking asylum

Refugees are people who have fled war, violence, conflict, or persecution and have crossed an international border to find safety in another country (UNHCR (UK), no date). People seeking asylum have left their country and applied for protection as a refugee. As stated by the UK Government, seeking asylum is a claim by a person to be recognised as a refugee under the 1951 Refugee Convention on the basis that it would be contrary to the United Kingdom's obligations under the Refugee Convention for them to be removed from or required to leave the United Kingdom. A person seeking asylum is waiting to hear the outcome of their application, and as such they have not yet been granted status as a refugee, as they have not yet been determined to have met the criteria for refugee status and permanent protection in the host country. People from these groups are at a higher risk of not having their healthcare needs met, and to have an appreciation of why and how perhaps the assessment tools that are used in practice may not capture all the needs of people from these groups is key to you being able to carry out a holistic assessment, to plan and give person-centred care. Some points for you to factor into the assessment process are that individuals from these groups have experienced forced migration and may well have experienced torture, religious persecution, sexual violence, loss of close family members, and living in refugee camps. Their journey to a safe country may have been dangerous and traumatic. Major et al. (2017) have identified that forced migration has disproportionate health, social, and economic burdens making the healthcare of people from these groups highly complex. Barriers to healthcare that exist for this group at an individual level may be language, communication, and cultural differences; an unfamiliar health system (Robertshaw et al., 2017).

Dr Jean Watson, an American nursing theorist who has written extensively on the theory of nursing and the theory of caring (Watson, 1988), talks about nursing being defined by caring. Watson's caring theory focuses on the relational processes that healthcare workers engage with patients' families and each other. In her theory of caring it is core that humans are not treated as objects and that humans cannot be separated from self, other, nature, and the larger workforce (Watson, 2008). Emphasis is on the interpersonal process between the caregiver and the care recipient. Dr Jean Watson's theories on nursing and caring capture the issues that have been discussed so far about the attitude of the nurse and the perception of the patient and their family about health and illness.

Recognising the diverse nature of the users of the health service is the first step. Then understanding their needs should follow to develop the relationship value, and this understanding of needs must be taken into consideration for care to be person-alised. However, given the wide range of diverse groups of patients, it is not possible to have an understanding of every diverse group and their cultural practices; there-fore, it should be the approach to diversity and cultural differences that is key. When undertaking patient assessment, the outcome is to understand what the patient's needs are. These needs are unique to the patient and will include clinical symptoms that need medical/nursing attention and issues specific to the individual that can affect their care.

When undertaking patient assessment, it is important for you to be prepared to address not just the clinical symptoms, but also the spectrum of demographics and personal characteristics that will influence individual beliefs and responses to health and illness. In Activity 5.2, you should have identified cultural data in the scenarios that are part of the spectrum of demographics and personal characteristics. Williamson and Harrison (2010) identify two approaches to defining culture and providing appropriate care, which can be considered as patient assessment in delivering care. Considering that it is an expectation to provide culturally appropriate care, one approach identified is a cognitive approach that focuses on cognitive aspects of culture, traditions, values, and beliefs with the assumption that they are shared by those from the same background or group. If this approach is used, it means that you would have to learn about specific cultural groups in relation to these cognitive aspects of culture to be able to assess and provide appropriate care. In addition, with this approach, awareness of your own cul-ture and being able to understand and accept difference is required. Learning as much as you can about how others see health and illness from their perspective may make you more sensitive to the individual needs of people from certain groups. However, the downside to acceptance that culture is something static and that all people who subscribe to that culture are the same is that this can lead to stereotyping. From your understanding of culture in the earlier chapters, there are differences within cultures, and people do change as they are influenced by other factors that change or adapt their traditions, values, and beliefs. The second approach suggested by Williamson and Harrison (2010) is a broader approach. Rather than focusing on cognitive aspects of culture as in learning about customs and beliefs of particular groups to plan appropriate care, the focus is on the individual's social position and how this impacts their health and well-being. This is a more critical approach. The reason why a more critical approach may be appropriate is that it provides insights into the social position and power relationships between the individual and how these influences impact on health. It includes, and is not restricted to, age, gender, sexual orientation, ethnicity, or migrant experience, religious/spiritual beliefs, socio-economic status, and disability.

# Cultural competency

Platform 3, 'Assessing needs and planning care' (NMC, 2018a), states that the registered nurse should work in partnership with people to develop person-centred care plans that take into account their circumstances, characteristics, and preferences. The process for this would start with patient assessment, and during this process you will need to develop the ability to collect relevant data about the presenting problem, which would include objective and subjective data. As part of the data collection to ensure that assessment and planning of care is clinically safe and culturally sensitive, relevant cultural data regarding the problem will be required, and you will need to develop the ability to extract this information from the individual and their family where applicable. For you to do this, you need to be culturally competent, bearing in mind that culture is not only about beliefs and values on race and ethnicity, but that other determinants, such as age, gender, education, religion, socio-economic status, and occupation need to be considered.

There are five attributes that define cultural competence which should be demonstrated by nurses during care delivery: cultural awareness, cultural sensitivity, cultural knowledge, cultural skill, and dynamic process.

## Cultural awareness

Cultural awareness should have emerged from the reflective exercise. In summary, this is about the nurse having self-awareness of their own cultural values, beliefs, and practices to better understand the practices of other cultural groups, and where personal stereotypes, biases, or assumptions are evident towards other cultures that are seen as different, recognising that these must be explored. Thus, within cultural awareness, the nurse becomes mindful of the different values, beliefs, norms, and lifestyles of the individual person and their family where applicable, recognising cultural similarities and differences, as well as the influence of culture on health and its value in nursing care provision.

# Cultural sensitivity

Cultural sensitivity is the awareness not to assume that individuals from the same culture are the same, as there is diversity within cultures. Appreciation of this diversity is key to achieving mutual learning and developing trust, as well as respecting cultural differences to allow genuine and satisfactory care.

# Cultural knowledge

Cultural knowledge is when the nurse has accomplished an educational base to better understand different beliefs, values, and behaviours of various cultural groups that they may be presented with in professional practice. Within cultural knowledge, the nurse will know about what are acceptable and unacceptable behaviours when interacting with different cultures in relation to etiquette, communication, and diet, to name a few activities. Having this knowledge and understanding when assessing and planning care better prepares the nurse before the encounter. It also means that a better service provision can be achieved.

# Cultural skill

Cultural skill is about the ability of the nurse to undertake a cultural assessment that collects relevant cultural data on the current health problem of the individual in a sensitive manner and to incorporate this data into the planning of care accurately. One of the key skills required is effective communication, which is addressed in Chapter 3.

# Dynamic process

Dynamic process is about 'becoming culturally competent' as a nurse rather than 'being culturally competent'. As identified earlier in this chapter, it is not possible for the nurse to know about all cultures and the diversity within those cultures. Globalisation and migration mean that nurses will continue to encounter individuals with different cultures from diverse backgrounds. Within these consistent encounters, cultural competence will gradually develop as the striving to provide care continues. Also, cultures change, and people change, and as such cultural competence cannot be a static process where there is no room for ongoing development.

Reflecting back on the previous scenarios, you should be able to see how a nurse can show cultural competence when assessing and managing events in the scenarios. The five attributes are areas that you should develop as you progress and transition throughout your nursing career. Having completed Activity 5.1, you can see that you may have some of these attributes already and can continue to develop those, or have identified that you do not have any as yet, but you now have a starting point to develop.

# Challenges in planning care for diverse patients

Having looked at the attributes when assessing and planning care in the context of culture and diversity, exploration of some of the difficulties you may encounter, as well as the causes, is also key. Look back to Activity 5.1, where you were asked to reflect on a clinical practice experience. The main areas of concern are stereotyping and labelling, as well as acculturation (Flowers, 2014).

Stereotyping is usually done unintentionally, and it involves making generalisations about some aspect of an individual or a group of people. However, not everyone in a specific cultural group has the same attitudes and assumptions about health and illness. As we have seen, there are various factors that can influence attitudes and assumptions when the focus is not on the cognitive aspects of culture. Within different groups, subcultures and variations exist, and just because a person may have the appearance that belongs to a certain culture, this does not necessarily mean they subscribe to what would be assumed as the 'norms' for that culture. Labels may be based on ethnicity, age, gender orientation, or disease.

Acculturation is another area that can pose challenges. There is an assumption that when an individual or their family has chosen to come to this country, they will integrate and adopt the British culture, modifying their own culture as a result of integration, and in some cases completely adopting British culture. This is not always the case, and there are many incidences where integration has not occurred and individuals have retained their cultural practices. In such incidences, it is important for the nurse to establish how much integration the individual and family have made to belong to British culture. Acculturation will be looked at again in Chapter 7 in relation to religious beliefs.

# Key points to remember when assessing a patient

Beliefs about health and illness will vary considerably between different cultures that you encounter and also within any given culture. Do not make assumptions, as looking the same does not mean being the same. There is a range of factors, including ethnicity and place of origin, education, religion, values, gender, age, family, and social status, that will influence the cultural perspective of the individual. As a nurse, when you undertake a patient's assessment and care planning, recognise that your beliefs and values about health for the individual and their family can be quite different from that of your patients. Even though it is possible that the same broad culture is shared, it is still important to value the individual.

To ensure that your assessment and the care you plan are culturally sensitive and meet the needs of the individual who has a different cultural background to yours, you will need to have an understanding of their perspective, which can be gained by asking more questions. The stereotype may not always fit; just because the individual looks different does not infer that they want to be different. Being culturally aware is one of the key steps you can take to start becoming 'culturally competent'. You can do this by recognising your own preconceptions that you may have when undertaking an assessment activity and aiming not to make assumptions, but instead seeking clarity and checking understanding from the individual and their family where relevant. The process is a lifelong learning activity as it is not possible to be knowledgeable about and understand all cultures and diverse groups. What you can have is an open attitude that *appreciates* the views of others, *behaviour* that validates and respects the cultural beliefs of others, and clear and open *communication* – the A, B, and C outlined by Heaslip (2015).

## Chapter summary

This chapter has given an overview of the impact of diverse cultural influences affecting one's health beliefs and the perception that illness has through reflection of your own beliefs about culture, diversity, health, and illness, allowing for the importance of assessing in the process of care delivery for patients from diverse backgrounds and communities.

# Activities: brief outline answers

## Activity 5.1   Teamworking (p90)

The ward manager getting the nurses together to discuss this was a good way to start addressing Martha's concerns with the team. Using the government position on care delivery as a starting point to remind staff how the team should deliver care to all patients was also an effective place to start. The NMC Code (2018b) or the Equality Act 2010 could also have been used. One of the simplest things they could do was to ask Martha how she wanted to be addressed as you would any patient and to respect this. Remember that Martha is a person and should be treated as such using individualised holistic care. Whatever uncomfortable feelings you have must be put aside. Transphobia is always unacceptable, particularly if it impacts on a safe assessment and care delivery.

## Activity 5.2   Critical thinking (p94)

### Scenario 5.2

This is about providing culturally sensitive care as everyone has a culture, and to assess and provide appropriate care the nurse must understand their culture, that of the profession, and be sensitive to the biases each individual or the family may bring to the therapeutic relationship.

In this case scenario, the health visitor did not fully understand the initial refusal of treatment by the family, and this would be an issue that they would have reflected on and discussed with colleagues as the family is not conforming to the 'norms' of care. When you then become culturally aware, the health visitor realises that their own personal beliefs and professional values of independence are the cause of upset with the parents' refusal to accept a referral to therapies.

The health visitor decides to go back and explore with the family their goals for their child. By doing this, they learn that the parents want the child to become stronger and have fewer infections. When the same therapies are described as a means of meeting these goals, the parents are quite willing to participate. The programme was developed to meet goals that the family identified as important.

In-depth knowledge of all cultures is unrealistic, but it is possible to gain a broad understanding of how culture affects beliefs and behaviours. Acquiring cultural knowledge begins with recognition that behaviours and responses viewed one way in one cultural context by the professional may have a different meaning in another cultural context for the individual.

## Scenario 5.3

When carrying out a patient assessment where the language barrier is an issue, an interpreter can be essential, as the nurse is responsible for assessing and understanding the information provided. It is important, as a nurse, to recognise the need for an interpreter, as illustrated in the scenario. Reliance on the child or other relative to interpret can be convenient for the parent; however, the nurse has to be sensitive to the needs of the mother and child. Given the nature of the presenting symptoms, both mother and son may feel uncomfortable talking about the current health issues, which may compromise the accuracy when taking the history. An interpreter, preferably female, should be quite urgently sought for the assessment to be thorough and accurate. The nurse will also need to address the child's concerns and fears in an appropriate manner. It would be an exceptional case if the child is used to interpret, and in cases where a family member is used to interpret, as a nurse, you must carefully evaluate each situation on an ongoing basis as you do not want the assessment to be inaccurate.

## Scenario 5.4

This is about working in partnership with the patient to develop a comprehensive plan of care that is individual and inclusive of the influence of the patient's culture and other influencing factors, such as family dynamics and roles within the family. In this scenario, the nurse has made an assumption about family dynamics, assuming that the partner is male and the mother is supportive of the entire family. The issue of family, even with current laws and openness, can be sensitive for many couples who are LGBTQIA+. For some, 'family' is often their chosen 'family' as opposed to their bloodline. Use of the word 'partner' and asking the patient who they wish to choose for a family meeting will show openness and a non-judgemental attitude from the nurse.

## Scenario 5.5

The focus of this scenario is on establishing mutual goals and being creative with a commitment to client-focused care, which are key attributes relevant to integrating cultural preferences into the plan of care. This is known as culture care preservation (Leininger, 1988). Having assessed the wound and taken into consideration Errol's preference, the nurse will have to consider the risk of harm depending on the nature of damage the wound has caused, as the nurse will have to decide if further input is required to manage the wound. Although the request is unusual, it does not pose any threat if appropriately cleansed and wrapped in gauze, as it will not be going directly on the wound surface, and the spiritual benefit of the relic to Errol should be recognised.

It is important for physical, emotional, and spiritual health to be able to integrate preference of the individual in the assessment and plan of care when there is no risk of harm to the individual or others. This does not mean that, as a nurse, you agree with or endorse the practice for the individual or for others.

## Scenario 5.6

This scenario is about the culture care re-patterning approach, whereby the nurse works with the patient to develop new approaches beyond the patient's normal way of doing things. In this case, the nurse needs to recognise that during times of crisis, such as ill health, a patient may revert to more traditional beliefs. This may differ from a choice taken prior to becoming ill and not following through fully. In this case, a sudden change in dietary practice has to be established. Having established this, the focus or goal is not to change Krishnan's beliefs, but to increase his choices and how to achieve adequate protein intake. It would be necessary, following assessment, to involve the dietician to teach him ways of how he can increase his protein intake from vegetarian sources. His spiritual needs should also be addressed by involving a Hindu priest; this is an effective way of addressing and providing him with insight into resuming animal protein if he so chooses. Ultimately, though, the choice will be his.

## Activity 5.3 Critical thinking (p94)

1. Role of family (roles of members, hierarchy, key decision-maker)

2. Role of the wider community with which they associate

3. Religion (impact on diet, beliefs about illness, treatment)

4. Personal views on health and wellness

5. Personal views on death and dying

6. Eastern/Western/alternative/traditional medicine

7. Beliefs about causes and treatments of illness, disease (physical and mental)

8. Gender roles and relationships and position within society

9. Sexuality, fertility, and childbirth

10. Food beliefs and diet

11. Socio-economic factors or status

12. Level of education

## Further reading

**Baker, M** (2016) Detecting pressure damage in people with darkly pigmented skin. *Wound Essentials*, 11(1): 28–31.

A good practical guide on how to assess a patient with a darker skin tone.

**Catalano, JT** (2015) *Nursing Now! Today's Issues, Tomorrow's Trends*. Philadelphia: FA Davis.

Chapter 22 in this book has an American perspective, but does give a good insight into issues that impact on nursing globally.

**Oozageer Gunowa, N, Hutchinson, M, Brooke, J, and Jackson, D** (2018) Pressure injuries in people with darker skin tones: a literature review. *Journal of Clinical Nursing*, 27(17–18): 3266–75.

A comprehensive review of the evidence that is currently out there on this topic. A must-read.

**Papadopoulos, I** (2018) *Culturally Competent Compassion: A Guide for Healthcare Students and Practitioners*. London: Routledge.

This book gives a well-structured, up-to-date guide on culturally competent care that is well worth reading. Chapter 4, on health and illness in multicultural societies, is particularly useful.

## Useful website

Intercultural Education of Nurses and Health Professionals in Europe (IENE):

**http://ieneproject.eu/mooc.php**

This multilingual website addresses nurses and healthcare professionals working in contact with patients of different cultures and languages, and aims to improve the quality of vocational education and training of nurses in Europe.

# Chapter 6

# Spirituality, death, grief, and loss

*Beverley Brathwaite*

## NMC Future Nurse: Standards of Proficiency for Registered Nurses

This chapter will address the following platforms and proficiencies:

**Platform 2: Promoting health and preventing ill health**

2.10 provide information in accessible ways to help people understand and make decisions about their health, life choices, illness, and care.

**Platform 3: Assessing needs and planning care**

3.4 understand and apply a person-centred approach to nursing care, demonstrating shared assessment, planning, decision-making, and goal setting when working with people, their families, communities, and populations of all ages.

3.14 identify and assess the needs of people and families for care at the end of life, including requirements for palliative care and decision-making related to their treatment and care preferences.

3.16 demonstrate knowledge of when and how to refer people safely to other professionals or services for clinical intervention or support.

**Platform 4: Providing and evaluating care**

4.4 demonstrate the knowledge and skills required to support people with commonly encountered mental health, behavioural, cognitive, and learning challenges, and act as a role model for others in providing high-quality nursing interventions to meet people's needs.

## Chapter aims

After reading this chapter, you will be able to:

• demonstrate what death means to different communities in the UK and how to support patients;

- demonstrate an awareness of the differences and commonalities between spirituality and religion;
- understand the needs of end-of-life care for diverse patients;
- identify the experiences of death, grief, and loss from differing religious and cultural perspectives; and
- look at how, as healthcare professionals, we use religion and spirituality appropriately in care delivery.

# Introduction

## Case study: imposing religious beliefs

A nurse at a Kent hospital was dismissed and then placed under restrictions for imposing her religious beliefs on patients, and in particular, giving her personal Bible to a patient. The nurse argued that she hadn't intended to impose her beliefs, and after a hearing at the NMC in 2018 the restrictions were lifted, and she is now able to practice unrestricted. She said, 'I didn't expect to be sacked so I was shocked. This means so much to me because I can go back to the profession I love.'

(Adapted from BBC News, 2018)

This unfortunate situation highlights how the best religious intentions can lead to significant penalties for a registered nurse. There are many positions that can be taken regarding what took place and the initial and final outcome for the registered nurse in the case study; here, the focus is on religion and the nurse–patient relationship. There was no malice intended by the nurse; she only wished to use her religion to help her patients. However, we are not all the same, and patients differ in how much they wish religion and spirituality to be incorporated into the care they receive. The RCN (2011) says *the nursing profession needs to explore and debate the boundaries that exist between personal belief and professional practice* (p5) and needs to be clear about how they express their beliefs in their own lives, whether through doctrine, ritual, or membership of a religious community. Such clarity is essential if they are to remain objective when assessing, planning, and delivering holistic patient care. This is supported by Clarridge (2017) and The Code 20.7 (NMC, 2018b), who state that nurses need to be aware of their own beliefs and values in order to best meet the spiritual care needs of patients, as well as the need for objectivity while providing support to the patient and not allowing their own values and beliefs to impinge upon or influence the patient in any way.

Moving away from personal interactions to healthcare more broadly, the following quotation addresses the varied perspectives that are out there about religion and healthcare:

> *There are many people who think religion is integral to health care. There are many others who think religion has no place in a healthcare setting. For some people, religion is a part of who they are and informs their decisions and actions. For others, it is something they want no part of – these people find it intrusive or even offensive to have spirituality or denominational religion introduced into health care.*

(Narrative Inquiry in Bioethics Editors, 2014, p189)

This chapter will look at these issues surrounding religion, healthcare professionals, and care delivery. We will discuss how the nurse practitioner must take into consideration the different religious faiths and spiritual needs of our diverse patients. The chapter will then discuss the complex concepts of religion, spirituality, and faith, and how they are combined into healthcare and nursing. Finally, we will examine how various communities view religion, death, grief, and end-of-life care, and how we, as healthcare professionals, can use their and our understanding of these issues to deliver high-quality care at one of the most sensitive times in a person's life journey.

## Religion, spirituality, and faith discussions in nursing and healthcare

According to the 2021 census for England and Wales, the five largest religions are Christianity (46.2 per cent), Islam (6.5 per cent), Hinduism (1.7 per cent), Sikhism (0.9 per cent) and Judaism (0.5 per cent). In 2021, London was the most diverse region, with the highest proportion of people identifying themselves as Muslim, Buddhist, Hindu, and Jewish. The North East and North West had the highest proportion of Christians, and Wales had the highest proportion of people reporting no religion (ONS, 2022a). 'Religion', 'spirituality', 'faith', and 'belief' are terms used separately or in varied combinations in the literature and clinical practice. It is safe to say that trying to define them is particularly difficult, and what will be done here is an observation of the evidence base 'debate' around the meaning of these terms (Paul Victor and Treschuk, 2020). McSherry and Jamieson (2011) claim that, as nurses, we should question these terms to encourage a greater understanding of what they mean for the patient and for nursing as a profession when delivering care. Pesut (2016) argues that religious practices *inform* spiritual practices, and what makes them different is that they are practised separately from organised religion. Paul Victor and Treschuk (2020) identify that the term spirituality has more than 13 conceptual components and is different from religion and faith. They also go on to state

> *Spirituality can be a connection to God, nature, others, and surrounding. Spirituality is associated with quality and meaning in life. Conversely, religion is attributed to traditional values and practices related to a certain group of people or faith. Religion is guided by*

*tradition, rules, and culture. Religion is defined as a personal set or institutionalized system of religious attitudes, beliefs, and practices.*

(Paul Victor and Treschuk, 2020, p107)

In relation to nursing practice, spirituality can be a valuable component (Hawthorne and Gordan, 2020). It can aid a therapeutic open and honest relationship between you, your patient, and their families; thus it can be a positive addition to nursing practice (Hawthorne and Gordan, 2020).

Part 2 of the Equality Act 2006 defines *religion* as *any religion* and *belief* as *any religion or religious or philosophical belief,* as opposed to *any religion, religious belief or similar philosophical belief* (Burford et al., 2009, p8). Here, legislation highlights the difficult task of defining religion and amplifies the strong connection between religion and belief. Therefore, many people who have religious values, faith, and beliefs consider spirituality to be a personal construct that we all have. This is influenced by personal beliefs, value systems, within a cultural context (Lalani, 2020). This means that as nurses we must consider who our patients are and what spirituality means to them, which may be different to what healthcare professionals think it is, taking this into consideration from initial assessment to discharge.

Spirituality is more about how a person expresses their values or beliefs; as Timmins and Caldeira (2017b) suggest, someone might self-identify as 'religious', 'spiritual', 'both', or 'neither':

*Religion and spirituality may largely service the same psychological function and the different terms that people use themselves may be a matter of personal preference or style. Therefore, people call themselves religious and spiritual, religious but not spiritual, spiritual but not religious, neither spiritual nor religious, and, very interestingly, a hair-splitting blend of religious spirituality plus nonreligion.*

(p50)

These terms are regularly used interchangeably. The key point to acknowledge here is that many of your patients will believe in something, and this may be based on an organised religion or not, spirituality, faith, or a combination of these, but an acknowledgement of this as part of your assessment is necessary in order to give holistic care to your patient (Paul Victor and Treschuk, 2020).

## Diverse communities, religions, and spirituality

How, then, do we, as nurses, think about incorporating religion and spirituality in our patient care, with diverse religious beliefs and cultural preferences around care delivery? NHS Scotland Chaplaincy Services (2007) have seven standards that strategically outline how religious and spiritual needs can be addressed across healthcare systems, from access to services, education, and training, to staff support. They remain as relevant now as they did at the time of publication, especially after the impact of COVID-19 on death and dying in healthcare.

Activity 6.1 requires you to do two things: (1) look at the spirituality and religion discussion, specifically in relation to clinical practice and care; and (2) consider the importance of incorporating differing religious and cultural points of view and beliefs when caring for patients from diverse backgrounds.

---

## Activity 6.1   Critical thinking

Go to NHS Education for Scotland by following the below link.

www.nes.scot.nhs.uk/media/xzadagnc/spiritual-care-matters-an-introductory-resource-for-all-nhsscotland-staff.pdf

Look up 9. Spirituality, Equality, and Diversity. Focusing on your interaction with the patient, what key approaches should you bring into your own practice?

*An outline of what you might find is given at the end of this chapter.*

---

The importance of religious and spiritual care for our patients, as well as what can be done to assure that these needs for our patients are met, is outlined in the NHS Education for Scotland document *Spiritual Care Matters: An Introductory Resource for all NHS Scotland Staff* (NHS Education for Scotland, 2021). This is practical and helpful guidance on how you can incorporate good practice around religion and spirituality. We will now look at the discussion around healthcare, nursing, religion, and spirituality, with a focus on professional bodies.

## The Code (NMC, 2018b)

Evidently, spirituality is important to nursing and patient care, as it has been clearly articulated in the code of conduct for nursing. This does highlight that currently; spirituality takes precedence over religion in the current nursing establishment. However, religion has had a strong connection to nursing and healthcare from its beginning. Religious communities such as nuns cared for the sick, destitute, and dying. Then the formation of the National Health Service (NHS) witnessed a decline in these religious connections as health and welfare provision became state-controlled and secular (Ramezani et al., 2014).

Within the nursing literature, Ramezani et al. (2014) discuss ideas of spirituality focusing on enhancing patients' spiritual well-being. The emphasis is on patient-centred care and ensuring that, as nurses, we consider all aspects of the patient's experience of health in order to deliver high-quality nursing care.

The RCN surveyed its nursing members to discover what was happening out in practice and how nurses were engaging with spirituality and religion. What follows is a break-down of key points.

# The Royal College of Nursing spirituality survey: categories and aims

| |
|---|
| **Exploration and analysis** |
| Discover and explore RCN members' understanding of, and attitudes towards, the concepts of spirituality and spiritual care. |
| **Prevalence and practice** |
| Identify whether the spiritual needs of patients are recognised by RCN members in the delivery of nursing care. |
| **Education and training** |
| Establish whether RCN members feel that they receive sufficient education and training to enable them to effectively meet patients'/clients' spiritual needs. |
| **Religious belief and spirituality** |
| Explore the associations that may exist between religious belief and RCN members' understandings of spirituality and the provision of spiritual care. |

*Table 6.1*   The Royal College of Nursing spirituality survey

*Source:* RCN (2011, p6)

As you can see from this list the focus of the RCN's enquiry was to find out more about spirituality, but religion was also part of the survey, emphasising the connection between spirituality and religion. Over 4000 RCN members participated in the survey, and the results did identify some important points. In culturally and ethnically diverse, learning disability, and LGBTQIA+ communities, there is evidence that repeatedly shows these groups do not receive care equitably, and the findings here indicate what a large number of nurses consider to be important in providing care by identifying how spirituality guides them in their practice. Analysing the data, McSherry and Jamieson (2011) identified the following:

1.  *Spiritual care is an integral and fundamental aspect of nursing care which may be indistinguishable from psychosocial care.*

2.  *Spiritual care concerns the personal caring qualities and attributes of the nurse such as showing care, compassion, cheerfulness and kindness in their communication and interaction with patients.*

3.  *Respecting privacy and dignity and supporting individuals with their cultural and religious beliefs are central to the delivery of spiritual care.*

4.  *Nurses were aware of the need to refer to and involve the patients' own religious/spiritual leader if necessary.*

5.   *Nurses, chaplains, patients, family and friends and other health care professionals were responsible for providing spiritual care.*

6.   *Nurses do not feel that they have a monopoly with regard to spiritual care and they are also aware of the need to liaise and collaborate with other healthcare professionals such as chaplains to support patients in this area.*

(pp1761–62)

These findings indicate the importance that spirituality plays in key aspects of delivering quality nursing care. The COVID-19 pandemic has highlighted the importance of McSherry and Jamieson (2011) and the RCN (2011) findings, as caring for patients at the end of life without family members being physically present was hard for both loved ones and HCP. The increased rate at which patients were dying in hospital due to COVID-19 made achieving spiritual care extremely emotionally and physically difficult for all involved in the end-of-life process.

However, as important as spirituality is, nurses find it challenging to give spiritual care and understand it:

> *Spiritual care is the collection of practices and behaviours that are generally seen as aimed towards helping someone to find spiritual well-being so that they have the strength and resilience to cope with the crisis they are in.*

(Clarke, 2016, p312)

This is so important for nurses when looking after patients from diverse backgrounds. These highlighted findings indicate that nursing care can impact more significantly on these diverse communities. As previously discussed (see Chapters 1 and 2), evidence suggests that equity of treatment from healthcare professionals in these aspects of care delivery is poorer than with the general population.

However, it must not be underestimated how much religion has a symbiotic relationship with spirituality, and never more so than with patients from diverse religious and cultural backgrounds. Religion is central to the lives of many people of African and Caribbean descent in the UK, most particularly Christianity (Burrell, 2019). Pesut (2016) suggests that the separation between theories of religion and theories of spirituality does not help the day-to-day lives of nurses in practice. Like many aspects of health, there should be a multidisciplinary approach to meet the specific needs of the patient (McSherry and Jamieson, 2011; RCN, 2010). There needs to be an awareness on the part of nurses of diverse patients' religions, spirituality, faith and health beliefs, rituals, practices, and observances in all healthcare settings. Being alert to patients' beliefs is vital, because these can have a major bearing on their health, both physical and psychological, as well as treatment (Burrell, 2019; Timmins and Caldeira, 2017a).

Religion does not exist in a vacuum; it is socially and historically rooted in society and healthcare, changes over time, and has a powerful shared effect (Pesut, 2016; RCN, 2010).

The same can be said of the history of different ethnic and cultural communities in the UK. It can be easy to focus solely on Christianity as it remains the most popular religion in England and Wales (ONS, 2022c). However, this would miss out on religious practices of differing ethnicities and cultural communities, as well as the impact that religion has on healthcare decision-making, reaction to distress, and managing and internalising illness. Without this knowledge and understanding that comes from religion, nurses may find it challenging to provide spiritual care that is sympathetic to patients' values and beliefs (Pesut, 2016).

Think about your own religious, spiritual, or cultural background. These are not some separate parts of you, as a nurse. While you may share the same religion as a patient, this does not mean that you know what the patient wants or that they will necessarily share the same beliefs (Mendes, 2015). An acknowledgement and knowledge of your patient's religious, spiritual, and cultural beliefs is important, but it cannot be fully understood without accounting for their personal identity, class, and heritage. Continuing from this point, Mendes (2015) considers that it is the impact of culture and religion on the person, and how this influences their personal beliefs and behaviours, that is arguably more important than learning about different religions or cultures.

Here, I argue that knowing about the religious, spiritual, and cultural needs of your patient gives you a starting point in which to assess and ask those important questions needed to determine the best course of action for your patient, which is of paramount importance when we are dealing with their health needs, both physical and psychological.

So far, there has been a focus on how religion, spirituality, and belief impact on physical health and patients' needs. Next, we will spend some time focusing on mental health and religion, as the emotional and psychological well-being of our patients is as important as their physical well-being. The NMC Standards clearly state that promoting and improving 'mental, physical, behavioural and other health-related outcomes' is important (NMC, 2018a, p12). Also, there is an evidence base that demonstrates a strong link between physical and mental health. Oman and Thoresen (2005) suggest that physical health benefits from religion and can facilitate gains in mental health, such as better social relationships, coping ability, and health behaviours. There is a give-and-take relationship between physical and mental health. B&B people can find support from religion against the discrimination that exists in society and when facing a deadly virus such as COVID-19.

# Mental health and religion

As a healthcare professional who should deliver evidence-based care, this is a vital question. However, the answer to this question is by no means straightforward. First, in diverse communities, which we have discussed in this book, some have a disproportionately higher level of mental health problems compared to the general population:

*Learning disability – Between 25 and 40% of people with learning disabilities also experience mental health problems.*

(Foundation for People with Learning Disabilities, 2019)

*Black Asian minority ethnic (BAME) community – Generally considered to be at increased risk of poor mental health compared to the general white population. If you look at the BAME based on gender women of colour experience mental health issues more so than men.*

(Mental Health Foundation, 2016)

*People from ethnic minorities are less likely than their White British counterparts to have contacted their general practitioner (GP) about mental health concerns, to be prescribed antidepressants, or to be referred to specialist mental health services.*

(Codjoe et al., 2019, p225)

*Irish travellers account for less than 1% of the Irish population, they account for 10% of the national young adult male suicide.*

(Mackey et al., 2020)

*Gay and bisexual men – have higher risks of substance abuse, suicide, depression, and anxiety.*

(Lassiter et al., 2017)

Therefore, when caring for patients in diverse communities, it is important that you take into consideration the patient's mental health as well as their physical health. The Mental Health Foundation (2016) also highlighted that some healthcare professionals are less likely to diagnose a mental health condition in B&B groups and that some B&B members are less likely to seek help. These issues are discussed in more detail in Chapter 8.

Religion can provide comfort and help, and give meaning to a person's life, bringing a sense of unity to their experience of the world that can be altered due to severe stress or anxiety, and must not be undervalued.

The evidence on the effects of religion and spirituality on mental health is complex. We will look at some of the positive and negative impacts on the mental health of some of the diverse groups previously mentioned, as well as what part religion and spirituality play (Rosmarin et al., 2022).

In the LGBTQIA+ community, spirituality and religion can relate to lower levels of depression, suicide, stress, and post-traumatic stress (Lassiter et al., 2017). Religious connection has been found to be associated with positive affect, better quality of life, greater life satisfaction, and higher morale. The negative aspects have been that:

*religion, particularly negative religious coping (e.g. passive reliance on the sacred; feeling abandoned by the sacred and extrinsic religious orientation) and spirituality, to a lesser extent, have also been associated with poor mental health outcomes.*

(Lassiter et al., 2017, p2)

Haney and Rollock (2018) consider what it is about religion that can make it a useful part of managing mental health problems. One aspect is through social interactions that occur when meeting in a place of worship such as a church, synagogue, or temple. Hanney and Rollock (2018) also go on to consider the following reasons:

*three aspects of religiosity may explain the relationship between religion and the mental health outcomes that it predicts: (a) extrinsic factors, including religious activities and social support from a religious community; (b) intrinsic factors, such as private prayer or the ability to derive meaning from a religious perspective; and (c) religious doubt, the questioning or feeling of disconnection from religious belief that may undermine religious coping and other spiritual processes.*

(p2)

Research by Codjoe et al. (2019) shows that B&B service users think that a positive relationship with their religion is essential to wellness and is more important than a medically focused view of mental healthcare. In the Black African community in England, the largest concentration of African Christianity outside of Africa can be found in the Borough of Southwark in London (Codjoe et al., 2019). This again highlights the importance of religion in connection to diverse groups and mental health. Codjoe et al. (2019) also go on to state that the Church can be used to reach members of the Black African community in a way to highlight that having mental health issues is something that needs addressing, as well as the importance of getting help and using the mental health services available (Turner et al., 2018). Mental health diagnosis such as depression is as important as a physiological diagnosis such as diabetes; both require the appropriate intervention by a healthcare professional.

It is important to make a concentrated effort to appreciate each person for who they are, incorporating their ethnicity, culture, sexual orientation, learning disability, and religious and spiritual needs. As diverse as communities are, recognising the need to respect the diverse meaning systems of each person is vital (Starnino, 2016). In other words, you need to find out how everyone interprets their lives and their religious or spiritual needs. As Codjoe et al. (2019) suggest, as mental healthcare professionals (MHCPs) (but valuable to all HCPs), *sensitivity and understanding of differing cultural and religious beliefs and how these relate to knowledge, attitudes and behaviours towards mental health* is important (p225).

Religion, spirituality, and culture have a strong connection (Lalani, 2020); therefore, this concept is important for two reasons, particularly as we are focusing on groups that are culturally and religiously diverse. The first is that those who have immigrated from their country of birth to the UK may well hold on to cultural and religious beliefs as they would in their country of origin. However, second- or third-generation immigrants who have been more steeped in British culture may have different belief systems.

So, what does this all mean for you as a nurse? Being familiar with the religious, spiritual, and cultural beliefs of your patient is important. However, just as important is your ability to be aware that your patient's beliefs may not be as fixed to your understanding of that religion or culture due to acculturation. Clarifying the specific needs of your patient and acknowledging their cultural, religious, and spiritual needs is something you must do, as your knowledge of their cultural and religious needs may be insufficient to meet their needs.

# Death, diversity, culture, and nursing

Death is a part of life and is something that you will experience personally and professionally. It is arguably one of the most challenging aspects of being a nurse. We focus so much attention on what we can do to save or prolong life that death can seem like a failure. However, death will come to us all. Sometimes there is time to acclimatise to a pending death and other times there is no warning. It is our responsibility and even accountability, as a registered nurse, to assure that all patients take the journey of death in the most dignified and respectful way possible, endeavouring to meet each individual wish of how, when, and where death should take place and helping them make varied decisions at the end of life (Phillips et al., 2019). However, communities that share cultural and religious beliefs make sense of death in differing ways: *Religion, belief and spirituality are conceptual informants of how individuals experience death, dying and bereavement* (Pentaris, 2018, p116).

The South Asian population in the UK continues to be the largest ethnic minority group (ONS, 2022a). Venkatasalu (2017) identified that South Asians continue to follow their cultural values and beliefs on death, dying, and bereavement, such as wishing to die at home rather than at a hospital or hospice. As with some African cultures, Islamic tradition favours supporting the dying person's family by going to their home in large numbers and coming together to comfort the immediate family. In Islam, this is considered as Sunna (a practice of the Prophet Muhammad). Do not assume that certain ethnic groups always align with certain religions, because this is not the case. People of varied ethnicities, cultures, and nationalities practise Islam, and there are varied types of Islam as there are varied types of Christianity.

Informing the family about a patient death, preparing the dead patient, performing religious and spiritual practices, and supporting the dead patient's family can be challenging (Khalaf et al., 2018). What we will do here is address one of these areas: informing the family that their loved one has died. To help you with this difficult task of informing the family of a deceased patient on the phone, see Activity 6.2.

## Activity 6.2 Communication

........................................................................................................................

Watch the video on delivering the news of a death by telephone by following the below link.

www.sad.scot.nhs.uk/video-wall/

Breaking the news of a death can be particularly challenging for health and social care staff when circumstances require them to do it by telephone. This video aims to help professionals prepare for and undertake these conversations.

The video gives some useful advice on what should be said and how, which can be used for your future practice. As a member of the team, it may be your responsibility to make this call.

During the early stages of the COVID-19 pandemic, these types of conversations were even more difficult to have. People were unable to visit their loved ones in hospital due to social distancing and infection control practices that were put in place in the first year of the pandemic. Many religious and cultural practices around death were helpful in making people feel more emotionally able to manage their bereavement through the lockdowns. Fardin (2020) goes on to suggest that appreciating the religious and spiritual beliefs of COVID-19-infected patients can improve their calmness and well-being. However, some cultural and religious practices had to be modified during the lockdowns, such as the cleaning of the body by the male members of the family, which is practised in Islam.

In Western society, death can be seen as a failure, and maintaining life for as long as possible is the goal (Wilkins et al., 2010). Another feature of the early pandemic stages was in complete opposition to this position, due to the speed of death and the unprecedented number of older people dying in the first wave. The way in which HCP managed dying patients and their families when they were not allowed to visit in hospitals was to focus on ways to keep them informed of what was happening. Phone calls were used more than ever before, and phones and tablets to enable face-to-face contact. Lim et al. (2022) call this virtual care and most hospitals across the globe introduced virtual family visiting. There were various benefits and weaknesses of virtual care. Benefits include reduced patient psychological distress, enhanced staff morale, increased patient-centred care, and the quality of life for patients and their loved ones. Weaknesses included HCP accessibility to video calls, concern for security and privacy, and several patients and family members having trouble with videoconferencing capability or lack of access to virtual devices (Rose et al., 2021).

The use of virtual care became important, but the lack of consensual therapeutic touch from both family members and HCP was unsatisfactory, leaving the family and HCP feeling unable to care for the patient's needs. The use of personal protective equipment (PPE) impacted on all forms of communication, such as eye contact and facial expression, that are impossible or difficult to be seen fully due to face masks and shields, and touch due to gloves. Touch preferences vary across individuals, based on personal preference, ethnicity, and religious practices, and need to be delicately considered. However, touch conveys support, reassurance, care, and compassion, and is an important part of delivering holistic care, even more so when a patient is dying (While, 2021).

When confronting issues on death, religious perspectives can give a framework in which to formulate and grapple with what it is to be human, how death is a part of life, and what happens after death, even when your patient and you may no longer consider yourselves religious. For some, it can be an integral part of their culture and influence ideas and beliefs around death (Setta and Shemie, 2015).

In light of the discussion on death, when delivering care to a person at the end of life, being aware of cultural and religious needs of different communities is important, but, as you will see, determining what is right for the dying person and the people most important to them requires you to ask questions.

# End-of-life care in diverse communities

In light of what has been discussed so far, the necessity to recognise the needs of cultural, religious, and ethnic groups is important. However, those in our communities with specific needs, such as learning disabilities (LDs), require special attention in palliative care. Evidence consistently highlights that the end-of-life needs of patients with LDs are a real test to provide due to *disadvantaging issues and circumstances including difficulties with cognition, understanding, and communication, complexities in decision-making processes, high levels of co-morbidities and mental health issues, and complex social circumstance* (Tuffrey-Wijne et al., 2016, p447), and this is as unacceptable as it is with patients from other diverse groups. Nyatanga (2018) considers concentrating on the patient as a person rather than as a cultural being, asking questions about what the dying person's wishes are in a sensitive and respectful manner, and what you can do to help them. This may seem obvious, and this should be done for all patients; however, with patients who have a learning disability, that discussion may not be with the patients, but could be with carers, family members, or legal guardians. However, do not assume that having a LD means that the patient cannot participate in these important decision-making conversations around the end of life (Moro et al., 2017). It may be that you are uncertain and lack knowledge of both your own and others' cultural and religious differences, which can make conversations difficult.

Some understanding of what is meant by end of life is also needed. You may have considered it means imminent death, but this is not the case. End of life encompasses patients 'approaching the end of life' when they are likely to die within the next 12 months. This includes patients whose death is imminent (expected within a few hours or days) (GMC, 2022). It is vital to support not only the patient, but their family members and significant others, through this particularly sad time, when an advanced, progressive, incurable illness takes hold and the patient and families need support through the last phase of life and into bereavement (NHS Scotland, 2019).

It is our responsibility, as nurses, to work collaboratively with the patient and the family to ensure that death is managed with the utmost dignity and respect, as well as assuring the care needs of our patients are carried out. Different communities have religious, spiritual, and cultural needs that should be recognised and valued.

## Case study: Dave

Dave is an 85-year-old man with end-stage dementia, and is being looked after by his son, Elliot, and his wife Marion at their home. The GP knows the family well, as does the district nurse, who is your practice assessor (PA) on your community placement. The GP has reviewed Dave. His breathing has become laboured overnight, and assessment indicates that he has only a few days left to live. The family are understandably upset and want to do the best they can for Dave. You ask your PA if the family have any specific religious or spiritual needs that have been previously discussed.

What questions could your PA and you ask to best find out this information?

*Answers can be found at the end of this chapter.*

Marion, Dave's daughter-in-law, had been going to church. After the initial phase of the COVID-19 pandemic, Marion had found this helped her manage her feelings about Dave's worsening condition. Dave and Marion's relationship had become even closer since his dementia started to worsen. She says that she would talk to Dave about what was said at church and that she felt he gained some comfort from it, and she would like to ask the head of her church to come to the house and see Dave, which perhaps could help all the family deal with him dying.

The support that can be given by a religious leader has a place in end-of-life care that is valuable, whether that be from your patient or their family members' personal religious leader or organised through us, as nurses. The role of chaplaincy can be key. Chaplaincy is based on Christian traditions, but now Buddhists, imams, and rabbis, as well as vicars and priests, can fall under the term 'chaplaincy'. What they have in common is the ability to give religious and spiritual care, compassion, listening, and cultural understanding, particularly, but not exclusively, at the end of life and when the patient is dying (Sanford and Michon, 2019). The receiver of chaplaincy support does not need to be of a particular religion. The all-important emotional support that can be given through the chaplaincy service is of significance to all patients and family members (Hurley, 2018). However, do not think that your patient and their family members may not want to talk to you about their religious and spiritual needs, and that once referred to chaplaincy you do not need to do anything else. Evidence indicates otherwise, and that discussing the religious or spiritual aspects of death, dying, and treatment with their healthcare professional is also important; therefore, you need to be prepared for this conversation

(NHS Education for Scotland, 2021). Evidence has also shown that the awareness of what the chaplaincies' role encompasses can be lacking (Ma et al., 2022). The role of the chaplaincy service has also changed through the pandemic, with the use of online ways of communication such as digital face-to-face platforms and calling more. The chaplaincy service has still maintained a presence in hospital through the pandemic, but their role was and still can be devalued (Snowden, 2021). Therefore, you not only need to have conversations with the patient and family members, but it is also incumbent on you to know who and why you are referring to the chaplaincy service.

Burrell and Selman (2022) highlight the vulnerability of the B&B communities in dealing with death, bereavement, and funeral preparations throughout the pandemic, gaining control of this process and navigating through the restrictions that were in place, such as limited numbers being able to attend a funeral. Accessing bereavement support and having local knowledge of specialist services and palliative care teams should be information that you are familiar with in order to provide information that is meaningful and culturally appropriate.

## Chapter summary

First, it is important to state that many of the points raised here relate to all our patients who we meet daily in a variety of different clinical settings. The importance of communication, respect, dignity, and person-centred, individualised care within the context of religion, spirituality, death, and end-of-life care cannot be underestimated. All our patients deserve this. We all have different religious and spiritual beliefs, even when we do not consider ourselves religious, and to some extent this guides us as humans – and nurses.

That being said, the evidence strongly identifies that patients who are older, or who have a LD, and those of different religions and ethnicities than the predominant white Christian tradition in the UK, do not view death and end-of-life issues in the same way, and experience poor care around death and end-of-life care. The COVID-19 pandemic has highlighted this even more and proved challenging to healthcare professionals and the public alike in dealing with death and dying when lockdown restrictions were in place. Being able to ask the right question and having the knowledge required to do this aids better clinical decision-making for the patient in a sensitive and respectful manner. Without this, it will be tough to give the level of care that these and all our patients deserve around such sensitive issues.

## Activities: brief outline answers

### Activity 6.1   Critical thinking (p112)

Your place of work needs to have some guidance and come from a position of equality and diversity to enable you to consider spiritual care of the whole patient, being patient-focused.

## Case study: Dave (p121)

Nyatanga (2018) gives a comprehensive idea of the types of questions that could be asked and why. These have been modified here. Of course, not all need to be asked, and not all at the same time, but you can see that specific questions must be asked to get as much information as possible to assess the needs of your patient and their family and carers.

- How did you all manage through the lockdowns?
- Is there any faith leader that you would like to be involved or that we could arrange for you?
- Do you have any rituals/practices that I should be aware of in order to help at this time?
- Could you help me to understand what is worrying you (if you think there could be psychosocial issues) or bothering you about Dave and what is going on now (if you suspect physical issues such as pain)?
- Did Dave have any specific needs that he informed you of or that you think would be important to him?

These questions will allow you to address their concerns (agenda) first by understanding their priorities before you can offer the best support available/possible. Proactive caring involves asking your patient or close family members direct questions.

## Further reading

**Burnard, P and Gill, P** (2014) *Culture, Communication and Nursing.* London: Routledge.

This book provides helpful guidance on how to communicate in an effective and culturally sensitive way.

**Murgia, C, Notarnicola, I, Caruso, R. De Maria, M, Rocco, G, Stievano, A and Gobbens, R** (2022). Spirituality and religious diversity in nursing: a scoping review. *Healthcare,* 10(9): 1661.

This study gives a good examination of nurses' perceptions of spirituality in the context of the religious diversity of patients. The review of the literature, discussion, and relevance for practice are particularly helpful.

## Useful websites

Visiting someone who may die soon during COVID-19:

**www.mariecurie.org.uk/help/support/terminal-illness/preparing/visiting-dying-covid**

Here you can find the latest information to help you work out if you can visit, how to see someone safely, and what to do if you cannot be there in person at a patient home due to COVID-19. Note these issues are constantly changing and be sure that you follow national guidance as well.

An international non-governmental organisation focusing exclusively on hospice and palliative care development worldwide. They are a network of national and regional hospice and palliative care organisations.

WHO Key Facts: Palliative Care:

**www.who.int/news-room/fact-sheets/detail/palliative-care**

The World Health Organization addresses key issues relating to palliative care globally, looking at what is being done to improve end-of-life care.

WHO Definition of Palliative Care:

**www.who.int/cancer/palliative/definition/en/**

A definition of palliative care and ways in which to implement palliative care across the life span.

Marie Curie: What Are Palliative Care and End of Life Care?

**www.mariecurie.org.uk/help/support/diagnosed/recent-diagnosis/palliative-care-end-of-life-care**

NHS: What End of Life Care Involves:

**www.nhs.uk/conditions/end-of-life-care/what-it-involves-and-when-it-starts/**

This NHS website gives more definitions of terms, as well as what can be done and who can be involved in end-of-life care.

NHS Inform: Palliative Care:

**www.nhsinform.scot/care-support-and-rights/palliative-care**

Palliative care is about improving the quality of life of anyone facing a life-threatening condition. It includes physical, emotional, and spiritual care. This is a comprehensive look at symptom control, the conditions that can cause palliative care needs, practical help, planning for the future, and preparing for death and bereavement.

Age UK: End of Life Issues:

**www.ageuk.org.uk/information-advice/health-wellbeing/relationships-family/end-of-life-issues/**

Age UK: Coping with Bereavement:

**www.ageuk.org.uk/information-advice/health-wellbeing/relationships-family/bereavement/**

Both of these Age UK pages are useful in directing patients and their families to information on end-of-life care and coping with bereavement.

*NHS Education for Scotland: Spiritual Care Matters: An Introductory Resource for All NHS Scotland Staff.*

**www.nes.scot.nhs.uk/media/xzadagnc/spiritual-care-matters-an-introductory-resource-for-all-nhsscotland-staff.pdf**

This NHS Education for Scotland document gives practical and evidence-based information to support healthcare staff who are working with patients, carers, and families around religion, spirituality, bereavement, and end-of-life care.

# Chapter 7

# Public health: meeting the needs of diverse communities

*Gillian Craig and Caroline McGraw*

## NMC Future Nurse: Standards of Proficiency for Registered Nurses

This chapter will address the following platforms and proficiencies:

**Platform 2: Promoting health and preventing ill health**

2.2 demonstrate knowledge of epidemiology, demography, genomics, and the wider determinants of health, illness, and well-being and apply this to an understanding of global patterns of health and well-being outcomes.

2.3 understand the factors that may lead to inequalities in health outcomes.

2.12 protect health through understanding and applying the principles of infection prevention and control, including communicable disease surveillance and antimicrobial stewardship and resistance.

**Platform 5: Leading and managing nursing care and working in teams**

5.12 understand the mechanisms that can be used to influence organisational change and public policy, demonstrating the development of political awareness and skills.

**Platform 7: Coordinating care**

7.4 identify the implications of current health policy and future policy changes for nursing and other professions and understand the impact of policy changes on the delivery and coordination of care.

7.13 demonstrate an understanding of the importance of exercising political awareness throughout their career, to maximise the influence and effect of registered nursing on quality of care, patient safety, and cost-effectiveness.

## Chapter aims

After reading this chapter, you will be able to:

- describe the key principles of a public health approach;
- discuss the needs of diverse communities affected by communicable (e.g. COVID-19) and non-communicable (e.g. diabetes) diseases and the need for a public health preventative approach;
- appreciate the importance of tackling not only individual factors and health behaviours, but also systemic health inequalities, as part of a public health approach; and
- demonstrate an awareness of different policy contexts and how to influence policy to address health inequalities in diverse communities.

# Introduction

Public health is defined as *the art and science of preventing disease, prolonging life and promoting health through the organised efforts of society* (Acheson, 1988, p4). There is a range of approaches and interventions that aim to prevent disease and improve the health of the public. In this chapter, we discuss interventions at the individual and community level, such as screening and immunisation, and those aimed at the population level, including government legislation. The ban on smoking in public places, the 'stay at home' order, and other measures designed to restrict movement and social gatherings to reduce the spread of coronavirus2 (SARS-CoV-2) throughout the COVID-19 (Coronavirus Disease 2019) pandemic during 2020–2022 are also examples of population-level interventions.

The introduction of the NHS in 1948 was arguably one of the most significant public health interventions, paid for through taxation, with its principles of care for all regardless of need, and free at the point of access. Interventions can be universal, aimed at the wider population, or targeted at particular groups or communities who are at increased risk.

A public health approach is based on a set of principles, including: the focus on improving the health of the population; a role of government in achieving public health; an emphasis on prevention; the need to address the underlying social determinants of health that cause health inequalities; and, we might argue, the involvement of individuals and communities in the co-production of knowledge about their health and interventions designed to improve health and tackle health inequalities.

Over a century ago in the UK, the average life expectancy was 48.4 years for men and 54 years for women. By 2018, life expectancy in England at birth was 79.3 and 82.9, respectively (ONS, 2021b). These changes can be explained by improvements in public health measures, including sanitation, the introduction of safe drinking water, improvements in housing, better diet, and advances in medical science. Prior to the COVID-19 pandemic, non-communicable diseases (NCDs) such as cancer, stroke, and heart disease were the leading causes of death in older age groups (Fenton, 2016). Although people are living longer, they may be living more years in poorer health, and this is most marked in deprived areas. Poor people are living shorter lives and with disabling conditions (the Marmot Review, Marmot et al., 2010, 2020a). It is estimated that 15 million people in England are living with a long-term condition, such as diabetes or chronic obstructive pulmonary disease (COPD), and the likelihood of living with one or more disabling conditions is greater in older and deprived groups (The Kings Fund, 2015).

The Commission on the Social Determinants of Health (Health and Organization, 2008; WHO, 2008c; as introduced in Chapter 2) highlighted how individual life chances vary dramatically, including illness burden, and premature mortality, depending on the circumstances (social and economic) in which people are born, grow, work, live, and age, and 'inequities in power, money, and resources' (Marmot et al., 2020b, p3). Differences in life expectancy (discussed in Chapter 2) are particularly marked in diverse communities. Ten years on, an updated Marmot Review highlighted that the gains made in life expectancy had stalled and that the fall in life expectancy was most marked in the most deprived 10 per cent of areas. This fall in life expectancy was attributed to government policies, including austerity measures and cuts in government spending, which have disproportionately impacted poorer and diverse communities. This suggests an important role for nurses in developing policy and advocating for communities (see sections on how much should governments intervene and policy at the end of this chapter).

We know that people from non-white ethnic groups (e.g. Bangladeshi, Pakistani, Indian, and Caribbean groups) often experience worse health compared to those from white ethnic groups. Other groups also experience worse health and worse health outcomes compared to the rest of the population. These include refugees and those seeking asylum, undocumented migrants, people with a learning disability, homeless and prison populations, looked-after children, Gypsy and Traveller communities, sex workers, and some groups of people who identify as lesbian, gay, bisexual, trans, queer (or questioning), intersex, and asexual (LGBTQIA+).

The Public Health England Strategy 2020–2025 set out a vision to protect and improve the health of the public and reduce health inequalities (PHE, 2019). The vision set out ten priorities which aimed to ensure that the care healthcare professionals provide enables people to live healthier lives and is fairer and safer through a strengthened public health system. The priorities include a smoke-free society, and measures to promote a healthy diet and healthy weight, such as the anti-obesity strategy discussed later in the chapter. Other priorities include cleaner air, the best start in life, and better mental health.

Nurses and midwives across different fields of practice will contribute to public health in a variety of ways. The Nursing and Midwifery Council, for example, has developed standards of proficiency for specialist community public health nurses (NMC, 2004). These expect health visitors, school nurses, and occupational health nurses to search for health needs through surveillance and assessment of the population's health and well-being, including the analysis of data, identifying risk, and screening for disease. Nurses and midwives will create awareness of health needs in terms of the actions individuals and groups can take to improve their health and well-being. Nurses and midwives will be expected to appraise and influence policies affecting health and make recommendations for change to improve health and well-being. Finally, nurses and midwives will facilitate health-enhancing activities that promote and protect the population's health and well-being. They will be expected to apply leadership skills to manage people, projects, and resources to improve health and well-being (see the section on leadership and influencing policy later in the chapter).

In order to illustrate how some groups experience particular health risks and potentially worse health outcomes compared to the general population, we have selected a number of activities to illustrate health needs in diverse communities, and the corresponding public health approaches that nurses and midwives can adopt. These are provided throughout the chapter.

There is a tendency to blame individuals for their poor health or assume that poor health can be corrected through education and the provision of information, rather than address the underlying social determinants that cause ill health (e.g. poverty) and which limit people's ability to make healthy choices. In order to counter this, we highlight the role of systemic inequalities perpetuated through social, political, and economic institutions. Inequalities refer to the differences in the health status of communities and the term can be used to describe differences in the care people receive, including access to services and treatment (The Kings Fund, 2020). For example, services may provide a suboptimal response, including: poor care, lack of integration of health and social care, low practitioner awareness of risk in relation to culture and diversity, and health improvement policies that fail to reach diverse communities. People may be exposed to different risks by virtue of where they live, for example, air pollution, and poor-quality housing. These inequalities are unfairly distributed and are avoidable with the correct policies and actions from the government (see the section on policy and government intervention at the end of this chapter).

In this chapter, we will explore the transition from communicable diseases (CDs) as a major cause of death in the nineteenth century to NCDs as the major cause of preventable deaths in contemporary industrialised countries, and, in the light of the COVID-19 pandemic, we highlight the re-emergence of infectious diseases as a significant threat to global health (see scenario on changes in the causes of death in East London). This context provides a rationale for the need for public health prevention and your role as a nurse or midwife in promoting public health. We will look at different policies underpinning nursing and midwifery practice and how you can address inequalities, by influencing policy, in order to achieve good health for individuals, families, and communities.

## Scenario: changes in the causes of death in East London

Annie was born in Stepney, in East London (in the South East of England, UK), in November 1874. She was the youngest of five children born to Thomas and Margaret. Thomas worked as a coal porter and Margaret as a sack maker. The family shared a one-room dwelling. Annie died aged just 13 months. The cause of death was recorded as tuberculosis. Her death was registered by her father, who went on to register the deaths of Annie's twin brothers from the same cause the following year.

Florence was born in Poplar in East London in November 1948. She and her two sisters were the first generation of children in her family to all survive into adulthood. On leaving school aged 15 years, Florence worked at a local sugar refinery. She was diagnosed with COPD aged 55 and type 2 diabetes aged 58. Ill health forced Florence to retire in 1996. Her retirement was marked by repeated acute exacerbations of COPD and hyperglycaemia. She was admitted to hospital on her 70th birthday with community-acquired pneumonia. She died three days later. Florence was survived by her two sisters.

Milton was born in Bridgetown, Barbados, in December 1952. Aged 18 years, he saw an advertisement in the local paper for the London Transport recruitment scheme. He applied, and after a successful interview, written test and medical, left Barbados. On arrival in the UK, he settled in Stratford in East London and worked as a bus conductor and later as a bus driver. Like many of his colleagues, Milton initially planned to stay in the UK for five to ten years before returning to Barbados; however, various factors, including economic hardship and raising a family, led him to stay and work for London Transport for the next 50 years. He died from COVID-19 on 6 May 2020. Milton was aged 61 years at the time of his death.

# A changing demography in the UK

The UK has undergone significant demographic changes over the last century. Not only has the size of the population grown from 27 million in 1850 to just over 67 million in 2020 (ONS, 2021c), but Black and ethnic minority groups now comprise 12.9 per cent of the population and there are approximately 9.4 million migrants (ONS, 2018). The population is also ageing, with 18.2 per cent aged over 65. In 2019, just over 1 million people identified as lesbian, gay, or bisexual, representing 2.7 per cent of the population (ONS, 2021d). The Foundation for People with Learning Disabilities (2019) reports that 1.5 million people are living with a learning disability. About 58,000 people living in England and Wales identified themselves as Gypsy or Irish Traveller in the 2011 census (ONS, 2014), and 1 in every 200 people in the UK is homeless (Shelter, 2017). Moreover, 24 per cent of young homeless people identify as LGBTQIA+ and 77 per cent believe their experience of telling their parents (i.e. 'coming out') was the main reason (The Albert Kennedy Trust, 2021), illustrating the need for preventative strategies. The different health patterns and care needs of diverse communities will require nurses and midwives to have specialist skills and approaches to tackling health and social inequality given these groups are often underserved by mainstream services.

# Changing patterns of disease

In the early nineteenth century approximately 70–90 per cent of the urban populations in the US and Europe were infected by tuberculosis (TB), a bacterial infectious disease, and nearly half of these infections occurred in cities because of the ease of transmission in densely populated urban contexts, with poor standards of housing, overcrowding, and poor ventilation. The number of people reported to have TB in 1913 in England and Wales was 120,000 compared with 4125 in 2020 (UKHSA, 2021). Whereas in the nineteenth century TB affected the general population, in contemporary Britain it mainly affects those experiencing deprivation.

The decline in the incidence of TB in the UK in the twentieth century (the number of new cases in a given period) coincided with public health sanitary measures, the clearance of slum housing and improvements in standards of living (Gandy, 2003). The introduction of antibiotic treatment in the 1940s, and implementation of the BCG vaccination programme in secondary schools in the 1950s, accompanied the decline in the number of cases until a resurgence occurred in the 1980s, attributed to the global HIV-AIDS pandemic and increases in travel and migration. In the 1940s it was nurses who were seen as an at-risk occupational group for tuberculosis and were offered the BCG as early as 1949 (University of Warwick, n.d.). The importance of immunisation to protect healthcare staff and patients is a theme we return to later in this chapter in relation to COVID-19, and in Activity 7.4.

Although preventable and treatable with immunisation and antibiotics, the World Health Organisation (WHO) considers TB as the second leading infectious disease killer after COVID-19 (WHO, 2022b), due, in part, to health system failure, late diagnosis and access to treatment, co-infection with HIV, and strains of TB resistant to antibiotic treatment (see HIV discussed later in this chapter to understand some of the barriers to accessing services and the section on underserved populations).

Between 1915 and 1945 infections continued to be a leading cause of death, particularly in young children (ONS, 2017a). In the 1950s there were regular outbreaks of measles, rubella, and mumps. Polio and pneumonia were common. Mass vaccination programmes were responsible for the decline of many diseases and by 1956, all children were offered vaccinations against tuberculosis, measles, whooping cough, diphtheria, and polio. More recent outbreaks of measles in the UK, and parts of Europe, however, illustrate the importance of maintaining high levels of vaccination (see Activity 7.4).

In the 1980s, the UK experienced a new challenge as a result of the HIV-AIDS global pandemic caused by the human immunodeficiency virus. At that time there was no treatment for HIV-AIDS until the introduction of life-saving antiretrovirals (ARVs) in the mid-1990s.

Death rates were high in the early phase of the AIDS pandemic when stigma around the condition was prevalent. Today, although there is no cure for HIV, HIV prevention strategies, for example, the use of condoms, access to needle exchange programmes and pre-exposure prophylaxis (PrEP), prevention of mother-to-child transmission, early testing and diagnosis (including testing for co-infection with tuberculosis), and rapid initiation of ARV treatment and adherence support, means HIV infection has become a manageable, long-term condition for those in contact with HIV services (NICE, 2016). Globally there were approximately 40 million people living with HIV in 2020 with over two-thirds living in Africa, and 680,000 people died of HIV-related illnesses (WHO, 2021).

The twenty-first century has once again witnessed the devastating impact of infectious disease with the COVID-19 pandemic, presenting additional challenges for health systems, professionals, and the public's health, both nationally and globally. Moreover, the pandemic has shone a light on pre-existing social and economic inequalities, which have contributed to a high death toll from the coronavirus (Marmot, 2020b), providing further evidence of the need for nurses and midwives to address inequalities to protect the health of the most vulnerable. The concern about new public health threats prompted a re-organisation of Public Health England (PHE), established in 2013 to protect the health of the nation, into a new health protection agency: the UK Health Security Agency (UKHSA), with a specific remit for planning, preventing, and responding to external threats, including pandemics. Together with a new Office for Health Improvement and Disparities (OHID), which will be responsible for non-communicable diseases, these two organisations will be responsible for public health.

Some concern has been expressed about the naming of the OHID, which fails to include the term 'public health', and the more commonly used term, 'health inequalities', opting for the less politicised term, 'health disparities', which may also illustrate the more 'libertarian' ideals of the Conservative Government, which emphasise personal responsibility for health and managing risk, rather than government intervention in the lives of individuals (Scally, 2021). This non-interventionist stance has been dominant throughout much of the pandemic: for example, the reluctance of the government to introduce measures to mitigate the risk of infection in England, such as the wearing of face masks. The Prime Minister, Boris Johnson, was only able to introduce these measures in the winter of 2021 with the support of the Labour Party, due to the opposition from his own political party. By contrast, the other UK nations (e.g. Wales, Scotland, and Northern Ireland) took decisions independently to introduce prevention measures to protect the public. Although the government insisted its policy decisions were based on evidence and scientific opinion, the different approaches adopted across the four nations suggest that politics, rather than sound evidence, can influence policy (see the section on should governments intervene and the intervention ladder in Figure 7.2).

## Underserved populations and inclusion health

In recognition that groups may be underserved by health and social care services, a new field of practice has emerged called inclusion health. Inclusion health has been defined as *a service, research, and policy agenda that aims to prevent and redress health and social inequities among the most vulnerable and excluded populations* (Luchenski et al., 2018, p266).

Public Health England highlighted the importance of language in defining underserved populations, that is, those populations who do not access mainstream services:

> People in this population have previously been described as 'hard-to-reach': this description can imply an active withdrawal of people from services but the lived experience of many is that services simply do not map to their needs in terms of accessibility, acceptability or suitability. 'Under-served' more accurately describes the experience of the population and puts the onus on service commissioners and providers to design and deliver services appropriate to the needs of the population.

(PHE, 2017, p6)

Public health approaches that aim to include underserved populations are discussed in the scenarios later in this chapter.

# The changing epidemiology of disease: from communicable to non-communicable diseases

Epidemiology is the study of the number of people affected by a disease or health condition. It examines how often a disease occurs in different groups and may tell us about the reasons for these differences. It can provide us with information about trends, for example, how many people have died over the course of the COVID-19 pandemic. It can tell us about vaccine uptake to inform vaccine prioritisation and targeting initiatives in low-uptake and at-risk communities. Information can then be used to plan and evaluate initiatives to measure improvement in vaccine uptake. Epidemiology relies on the collection of robust data and is important in order to prevent disease and premature mortality.

Health professionals and the general public were provided with information about the epidemiology of the COVID-19 pandemic, for example, the number of people infected, hospitalised, and deaths, with comparisons between the four nations in the UK, and other global contexts, in daily briefings from the government and Chief Medical Officer between 16 March and 23 June 2021.

## COVID-19: an example of a communicable disease

The WHO declared the COVID-19 outbreak a pandemic in March 2020. As most Western governments struggled to contain the virus, scientists set to work to develop a vaccine and find treatments. The first human trials for a vaccine started in March 2020. Italy was the first European country to implement a nationwide lockdown in March 2020; the US declared a state of emergency and countries around the world began to close their borders to international travel to stop the spread of the virus (New Scientist, 2021).

The WHO has recorded over 627 million confirmed cases of coronavirus globally and over 6 million deaths (as of 1 November 2022), with the UK reporting nearly 24 million cases of infection and between 177,000 and 206,000 deaths (UKHSA, 2021). According to data provided by the Office of National Statistics (ONS, 2022a), the risk of death from COVID-19 was lower in those who were vaccinated (i.e. two doses 21 days before infection). COVID-19 had a disproportionate impact on the most deprived areas in England, where rates were almost double the least deprived in the first 12 months of the pandemic. Diabetes was the most common underlying condition, reported in almost a quarter of those who died (see the section on NCDs).

Common to many high-income countries was the number of deaths in older age groups in the social care sector in the first wave of the pandemic; a finding, in the UK at least, attributed to poor understanding and prioritisation of social care services relative to the NHS, a lack of representation from social care staff to advocate for older people on government advisory committees, and a lack of testing capacity and personal protective equipment (PPE) to help with infection control. Moreover, older people were rapidly discharged into care homes to increase the capacity of the NHS, but without adequate testing and isolation facilities; this allowed the infection to spread, resulting in a substantial number of avoidable deaths (House of Commons Health and Social Care, and Science and Technology Committee, 2021).

Other groups were also disproportionately impacted by either COVID-19 or the prevention measures used to control the pandemic. We will now examine how the pandemic shone a light on inequalities in England with respect to people with learning disabilities (LDs), Black and Minority Ethnic communities, and LGBTQIA+ communities.

## People with learning disabilities and COVID-19

Prior to the pandemic people with a learning disability experienced significant, and largely preventable, health, social, and economic inequalities. They were three times more likely to die, and to die sooner, compared to those without a learning disability; on average 14 and 18 years for men and women, respectively, and from conditions that could be avoided with good healthcare (Heslop et al., 2014); a consistent finding across many countries. They are also likely to experience multiple health conditions such as mental ill health, epilepsy, obesity, and diabetes (type 1 and type 2, NHS Digital, 2021); conditions which may make them more susceptible to COVID-19, including higher rates of mortality compared to the general population (Williamson et al., 2021).

People with a learning disability are more likely to experience poverty, a risk factor for poor health, and are less likely to have employment. They were significantly affected by the cuts in public sector funding, such as those witnessed during the austerity years (from 2008 onwards). One study suggested that 42 per cent of people reported they had lost care and support services, resulting in a reduction in daily activity (Forrester-Jones, 2020).

Approximately 40 per cent of people with a LD are not diagnosed in childhood and they are also more likely to spend time in custody compared to the general public (Rickard and Donkin, 2018). It has been estimated that half of the increased risk of poor mental health can be attributed to poverty, poor housing, bullying, and discrimination (Rickard and Donkin, 2016). Bullying, abuse, and mistreatment of people with a LD by care staff were brought to the public's attention through the Winterbourne View Hospital scandal. The Crown Prosecution Service treated this abuse as a disability hate crime and 11 care staff were convicted, with some sentenced to jail (Department of Health, 2012).

In addition to poor-quality health and social care services, inadequate policy responses also reinforce inequalities. For example, during the COVID-19 pandemic, a blanket application of 'Do Not Resuscitate' orders (DNRCPRs) unlawfully targeted people with a LD and would have increased the risk of death for those infected with COVID-19. Some care homes received letters stating that, as people were unlikely to be admitted to hospital due to pressure on intensive care beds, DNRCPR forms should be signed for those who lacked mental capacity (Thomas, 2020). Undoubtedly this policy aimed to prevent the NHS from becoming overwhelmed, but highlighted how the most vulnerable were negatively impacted by the policy in the early phases of the COVID-19 pandemic. Similarly, some authors have argued that the emphasis on shielding, testing, and PPE in the early days of the pandemic contributed to loneliness and isolation. This example illustrates how policies aimed at the general population can negatively impact people with LDs, an issue explored in an activity later in this chapter.

COVID-19 therefore severely impacted a group that was already experiencing significant health, social, and economic inequalities. The result was higher rates of hospital admission and death. In England, the death rate from COVID-19 has been estimated as six times higher for people with LDs than the general population and 30 times greater amongst younger adults, aged 18–30. Those living in residential care, where a third of all deaths of people with a LD occurred, were particularly affected in the Spring of 2020 (PHE, 2020b). COVID-19 was able to exploit systematic, structural inequalities, and pandemic prevention policies may have inadvertently contributed to social isolation and the withdrawal of support services as all resources were redirected towards pandemic prevention.

## Racially minoritised communities and COVID-19

In this chapter, we use the term *racially minoritised* to refer to non-white communities, rather than the acronym BAME (Black, Asian, and Minority Ethnic). By using this language we aim to highlight that health inequalities arise as a result of social structures and social processes (e.g. racism and social and economic discrimination); these social determinants can help to explain the differential outcomes in COVID-19 and other health conditions (Milner and Jumbe, 2020).

The COVID-19 pandemic had a disproportionate effect on racially minoritised people who experienced higher rates of infection and mortality compared with their white peers. Health and social care staff from these communities were also impacted. For example, 50 per cent of NHS staff who died of COVID-19 were born outside the UK (DHSC, 2020).

In order to explain these differences, The Kings Fund (2021) reported that living arrangements (overcrowded housing), underlying health conditions (higher rates of cardiovascular disease, diabetes), socio-economic deprivation, geography, and occupation (i.e. those working in occupations with direct contact with the public increasing exposure to COVID-19) accounted for the excess mortality. The lack of culturally sensitive public health communication, tailored to the needs of different racially minoritised communities, may also have contributed.

# LGBTQIA+ communities and COVID-19

*LGBTQ communities are always disproportionately affected in institutions, structures and crises because they have a different set of needs.*

(Wareham, 2021)

LGBTQIA+ communities are another group that experience significant disadvantages, health inequalities, and unmet needs, and these were exacerbated during the pandemic. For example, prior to the pandemic LGBTQIA+ people were more likely to experience poor mental health, and were more likely to smoke, drink, use drugs, and report that they feared discrimination from health services (Stonewall, 2018). The LGBT Foundation (2020) conducted an online survey in 2020 which aimed to scope the experience of the pandemic on the lives of the LGBTQIA+ community, feeling this information was missing from the general COVID-19 narrative. During the lockdown LGBTQIA+ communities, in particular, found themselves separated from supportive and 'identity-affirming' safe spaces (Wareham, 2021). A key finding of the survey was the need for support for mental health (42 per cent), which increased to 66 per cent for respondents from racially minoritised LGBTQIA+ communities, 48 per cent of disabled LGBTQIA+ people, and 57 per cent of trans people. Some LGBTQIA+ people (8 per cent) reported that they did not feel safe where they lived, which illustrates how 'stay-at-home' orders can negatively impact diverse communities. Just under a fifth (16 per cent) had been unable to access healthcare for non-COVID-19-related issues.

A European survey, reported by NAM Aidsmap (Cairns, 2021), examined the effects of the pandemic on HIV care, and highlighted a marked reduction in HIV prevention and testing services across many countries; that is, services either closed completely or were reduced by half. Nearly a third of countries reported that they had reduced their outreach services by half as resources were redirected towards fighting the pandemic. Where services maintained appointments, these were offered through telemedicine, which could worsen digital inequality for those with poor access to the internet, or for those lacking privacy and with concerns about confidentiality.

# Vaccine hesitancy, inequity, and access

The COVID-19 vaccination programme began in December 2020 and in December 2021, the government announced an ambitious programme of offering a million vaccines per day as part of a booster vaccination campaign to protect against the effects of the Omicron variant of SARS-CoV-2, which dominated the UK.

The WHO set a target of 70 per cent of global vaccination coverage by the middle of 2022, but only 58 out of 194 member states achieved this target and just over a third of healthcare workers had received their primary vaccination.

Vaccine hesitancy is one barrier to people accessing the vaccine programme. The term vaccine hesitancy refers to: *a delay in acceptance or refusal of vaccines despite the availability of vaccine services* (Butler, 2022; Razai et al., 2021). The Office for National Statistics (ONS, 2021b), based on data from its Opinion and Lifestyle Survey conducted in the earlier part of 2021, reported that people from racially minoritised communities (namely Black or Black British), unemployed people, and those from deprived areas were most hesitant towards vaccines across all UK regions. Vaccine hesitancy amongst the health and social care workforce was also of concern; however, the policy of mandatory vaccination as a condition of employment for healthcare staff with direct face-to-face, patient contact was abandoned because of opposition from medical bodies fearing the impact on staffing levels if workers left the NHS (see the section on whether vaccination should be made mandatory later in the chapter. Activity 7.4 invites you to reflect on your views about mandatory vaccination).

Low uptake of vaccines in pregnant women was also of concern: misinformation based on rumours about the impact of the vaccine on fertility and menstruation was seen to play a role in vaccine hesitancy and concerns about safety. However, one research study found that unvaccinated pregnant women had a greater need for hospital treatment compared to vaccinated women; for example, 98 per cent of 1714 of admissions (Iacobucci, 2021). COVID-19 may also adversely affect the unborn child; mothers who tested positive for the virus at the time of birth were more likely to need a caesarean section, have pre-eclampsia, and were twice as likely to have a stillbirth, while one in five had a premature baby (Iacobucci, 2021).

NHS England and NHS Improvement identified two main ways to address inequality in vaccine uptake: outreach and information and education using a variety of media. Examples of initiatives to outreach services into the community to make the vaccine more available and increase vaccine uptake include: walk-in vaccination services where no appointment is required, and pop-up vaccination clinics in mosques and churches to access faith and local communities, shopping centres ('shots while you shop'), football stadia (e.g. the 'Gunner get jabbed' campaign in partnership with Arsenal Football Club at the Emirates Stadium, London, UK), schools, community centres, and community pharmacists offering open access clinics. Some countries developed innovative approaches to help people manage vaccine anxiety. In the Netherlands, for example, some clinics used virtual reality technology, including headsets, to counter people's fear of needles.

## Diabetes: an example of a non-communicable disease

Globally, NCDs account for approximately 70 per cent of mortality (Vos et al., 2020). In 2016, there were 533,100 deaths from NCDs in the UK (WHO, 2018). These included: cardiovascular disease, cancer, respiratory diseases (e.g. COPD), and diabetes. While NCDs are often viewed as separate from infectious diseases, the current coronavirus pandemic has highlighted the connection between communicable and non-communicable diseases as evidence shows that people with NCDs are at increased risk of becoming severely ill with the coronavirus. Furthermore, the pandemic curtailed the provision of health services for people with NCDs, including reductions in screening, detection, and treatment services (WHO, 2020).

Tobacco use, unhealthy diet, physical inactivity, and harmful use of alcohol increase the risk of NCDs. As such, these conditions are sometimes referred to as 'lifestyle-related diseases'. However, as we illustrate in relation to food environments at the end of the chapter, healthy food choices are often determined by factors other than individual choice. Addressing the needs of people living with NCDs is critical to not only reducing the risk of disability and premature deaths in ordinary times, but also to help lessen the impact of COVID-19 and enhance protection against future pandemics.

Diabetes is one of the most common NCDs and an important public health problem. If it is not well managed, it can cause serious health problems, disability, and early death. According to Diabetes UK (2021), diagnosis of diabetes has doubled over the past 15 years, and there are currently approximately 4.1 million people in the UK who have either type 1 diabetes (T1D) or type 2 diabetes (T2D). Around 90 per cent of people with diabetes have T2D, of which key risk factors are: being overweight, abdominal obesity, physical inactivity and high blood pressure. The burden of T2D diabetes is not equitably distributed across society. The Kings Fund (2021) reported that South Asian groups are six times more likely to develop T2D than white groups, while the prevalence in Black groups is up to three times higher than in the white population. Both South Asian and Black groups have higher mortality from diabetes than the white population. The Kings Fund also found that South Asian groups with T2D have a higher risk of developing secondary complications, including cardiovascular disease and end-stage renal disease, while Black groups have a higher risk of hypertension and stroke, but less propensity to heart disease.

Another group experiencing high rates of diabetes is people with LDs. According to Public Health England (PHE, 2020a), the General Practice Extraction Survey for 2017/2018 found that 6.8 per cent of people with LDs have T2D compared with 4.5 per cent of the general population. They also reported that people with LDs develop T2D at an earlier age; for example, 6.7 per cent of people with LDs aged 35 to 44 years have T2D, compared to 1.8 per cent of people in the general population.

There are multiple factors that contribute to disparities in diabetes. At the individual level, these include biological factors, health behaviours, and early life events (Golden et al., 2012). Biological factors relate to differences in fat distribution, glucose metabolism, insulin resistance, and glycaemic control in different ethnic groups. Health behaviours include differences in physical activity, smoking, and self-monitoring of blood glucose. Early life events include prenatal undernutrition, maternal stress, and maternal obesity during pregnancy. These early life events highlight the importance of policies and interventions across the life span, including perinatal and maternal health, from conception to the first two years of life, and beyond.

While individual differences may go some way to account for the variations in diabetes prevalence and health outcomes, for people with diabetes the contribution of the wider social and structural determinants need to be considered. For example, a survey of barriers to people with diabetes accessing eye care services in eight countries identified cost, long waiting times for appointments, and length of wait in clinics once an appointment had been scheduled (International Diabetes Federation, 2020). Proximity to care was also a factor. Few people were enrolled on diabetes management programmes because they were either not available or people did not know about them. Furthermore, the role of structural racism and discrimination cannot be ignored (Golden, 2021).

There is evidence of direct discrimination in the provision of healthcare services. For example, Public Health England (PHE, 2020a) reported a recent national audit for England and Wales, and found that people with LDs and T2D were less likely to receive nationally recommended regular monitoring and surveillance, annual diabetes checks, and structured education compared to people with no learning disability. Under the Equality Act 2010, it is the legal responsibility of commissioners and providers of healthcare services to provide diabetes care that meets the extra needs of people with LDs. According to Diabetes UK (Diabetes UK, 2017), the key steps to ensuring diabetes services meet the needs of people with a LD are: making information accessible, providing training for staff, addressing social barriers, involving supporters, and planning for and making reasonable adjustments.

Culturally tailored diabetes prevention programmes are also recommended to ensure health messaging campaigns, and healthcare interventions, are appropriately designed for diverse communities to access them (Lagisetty et al., 2017). One framework that healthcare professionals can use to enhance their client relationship, and enable the development of interventions consistent with social differences and religious and cultural practices, is the 'social grraacceess' framework outlined in Chapter 3.

# From evidence to action: the role of the nurse and midwife in addressing health inequalities

In Chapter 2, you were introduced to the Marmot Review (Marmot et al., 2010). To recap, the Marmot Review recommended an evidence-based strategy to address health inequalities based on six policy objectives. These policy objectives recommended: giving every child the best start in life; enabling children, young people, and adults to maximise their capabilities and have control over their lives; creating fair employment and good work opportunities for everyone; ensuring a healthy standard of living for all; creating and developing healthy and sustainable places and communities; and strengthening the role and impact of ill health prevention.

The importance of giving every child the best start in life is because disadvantages – and advantages – are cumulative across the life span, resulting in sustained inequalities between communities that can have effects across generations. Failure to intervene early can have consequences in adult life. The Marmot policy objectives broadly inform the Public Health Outcomes Framework (PHOF). Introduced in 2012, and last updated in 2021, the PHOF provides data on a set of health and social indicators, known as the Marmot indicators, which help monitor trends in public health across four domains. These include actions to address: 1) the wider determinants of health, 2) health improvement, 3) health protection, and 4) healthcare, public health, and preventing premature mortality (see Figure 7.1).

The vision underpinning the PHOF is: *to improve and protect the nation's health and improve the health of the poorest fastest* (Office for Health Improvement and Disparities, 2021). The purpose of the framework is to tackle inequalities in healthy life expectancy across different communities. Each of the four domains incorporates a set of public health indicators which can be used as a benchmark to see how well local authorities are doing in tackling inequalities. To illustrate the role of the nurse and midwife, we have chosen a number of activities highlighting interventions, or models of care, that aim to improve practice, with an emphasis on diverse communities; these can be found throughout the chapter (see Figure 7.1).

# Health improvement for racially minoritised pregnant women through the provision of continuity of care by midwives and health visitors

A recent study highlighted how deprivation and ethnicity (both social determinants of health) are risk factors for adverse pregnancy outcomes. Researchers looked at the birth records of 132 NHS hospitals in England, between April and March 2017, to examine the effects of deprivation and ethnicity. They found that differences in socio-economic status (wealth) and ethnicity could explain the increased risk of stillbirth, preterm birth, and foetal-growth restrictions, and that these inequalities were most marked in the most deprived Black and South Asian groups (Jardine et al., 2021).

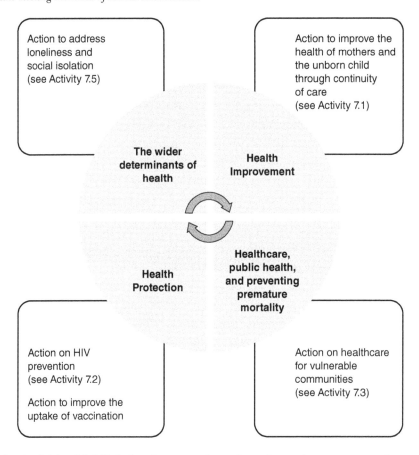

*Figure 7.1* Activities highlighting interventions that aim to improve practice

The research evidence confirms the importance of the first 1001 days, the period from conception to the age of 2 years, on the health, development, and achievement of children. Early intervention therefore can have an impact across the life span and help to address inequalities by giving every child the best start in life (Marmot et al., 2010).

The NHS plan set out a vision in 2021 that: *35% of all women should be on a continuity pathway with at least as many women from the BAME communities and the most deprived communities receiving continuity of care as white women.* There is also evidence to suggest that effective targeting of continuity of care to racially minoritised groups, and those living in deprived areas, can lead to improvements in clinical outcomes. Public Health England (PHE, 2021) has defined continuity of care as: *planned and sustained delivery of high-quality support and includes providing consistent messages, effective handover of care, joint working and good working relationships.* Public Health England (2021) also produced guidance on care continuity for midwives and health visitors. Activity 7.1 asks you to read this guidance and answer questions about the continuity of care.

## Activity 7.1   Critical thinking

Health visitors are qualified nurses or midwives who have completed a specialist community public health programme. Health visitors must offer every parent a minimum of five health and development reviews and meet with parents at 28 weeks for an antenatal review. They are required to meet with parents at specified time intervals after a baby's birth up to two and a half years of age. Read the Executive Summary of the guidance on continuity of care produced by Public Health England (2021) and answer the following questions:

- Why is continuity of care important?
- What factors can contribute to health visitors and midwives working together effectively to provide continuity of care?
- How has the COVID-19 pandemic impacted the work of professionals to provide continuity of care?

*Because the answers are provided in the Executive Summary, there is no outline answer provided at the end of this chapter.*

# Health protection: innovative service models for providing pre-exposure prophylaxis (PrEP) to prevent HIV infection

Globally there were 37.7 million people living with HIV in 2020 with over two-thirds living in Africa, and 680,000 people died of HIV-related illnesses (WHO, 2022a). Approximately 105,000 people were living with HIV in the UK in 2019 and 41 per cent of all new HIV diagnoses were in men who have sex with men (MSM), including gay, bisexual, and other men. Trans women are also at risk of acquiring HIV through sex between men. Delays in diagnosis, however, remain the greatest threat to prevention and treatment, and in the UK approximately one in every 16 people infected with HIV remains undiagnosed despite the availability of rapid diagnostic testing with same-day results (National AIDS Trust, 2021).

Black African people make up 18 per cent of all new diagnoses of HIV and in 2019 nearly half of these were late diagnoses, suggesting there are barriers to getting tested and accessing care. These include: cultural and structural racism, shame, fear of stigma and discrimination, poor access to culturally and gender-sensitive services, and low awareness of personal risk and how to access preventative care. For example, PrEP is medicine people can take to prevent getting HIV through sex or injecting drug use, but awareness of PrEP, and its uptake in Black African communities (amongst men and women), is low compared to gay and bisexual men, despite making up 44 per cent of new heterosexual HIV diagnoses (Terrence Higgins Trust, 2019).

Activity 7.2 asks you to think about the barriers to accessing care and how different service delivery models could improve uptake based on examples from the global context.

## Activity 7.2    Critical thinking

PrEP is a medication used to reduce the risk of getting HIV and is recommended for those who are HIV-negative but at risk of HIV infection, for example, those with a partner with HIV. It is currently available in England, Scotland, and Wales, free of charge, through sexual health clinics. However, some members of the LGBTQIA+ (e.g. trans women) and racially minoritised communities may experience specific barriers to accessing PrEP through sexual health clinics. What are these barriers and what lessons can we learn about how to improve access based on models of care in the global context?

*An outline answer is not provided as you can find out this information in the link to a summary of different models of PrEP designed to increase access, produced by NAM AIDSMAP:* www.aidsmap.com/news/jan-2019/six-innovative-models-prep-services

# Healthcare, public health, and preventing premature mortality

Public health pandemic prevention measures, which aimed to protect the general public, impacted negatively on many diverse communities because they were already experiencing disadvantages due to systemic inequalities, and both the pandemic, and measures to counter the pandemic, were able to exploit these. Sex workers, for example, were not able to work due to restrictions on interactions with people outside an individual's household in the earlier phase of the pandemic, and they were not eligible for government support for self-employed people because of the lack of formal documentation, such as tax records. This may have pushed sex workers to engage in high-risk behaviour to compensate financially (Mergenthaler and Yasseri, 2021). Whereas the needs of sex workers were overlooked at the start of the pandemic, the government more proactively aimed to protect homeless populations by offering temporary accommodation in hotels. This not only helped to stop the spread of infection but provided an opportunity to improve the health of some groups of homeless people.

## Activity 7.3    Communication

Read the article on how nurses worked to improve the health of homeless people, drawing on the experiences of Rosa Ungpakorn, who won an RCNi Advanced Nurse Practitioner award for her homeless outreach activities. Discuss how these initiatives supported homeless people with your practice supervisors.

www.rcn.org.uk/magazines/bulletin/2020/june/homeless-health-nursing-during-covid-19-pandemic

*An outline answer is not provided as you are asked to read and discuss the information.*

# How much should governments intervene in the lives of citizens to protect the public's health?

Examples of government intervention to protect the health of citizens range from public health sanitary measures, introduced as a result of the Public Health Act in 1848, in response to the cholera epidemics, and the introduction of seat belts in the 1980s in the UK. Legislation was used to prevent smoking in enclosed spaces in 2007, and smoking in cars with children under the age of 18 was also banned in 2015 to protect them from the harm of second-hand smoke. Governments have therefore increasingly intervened in the domestic sphere, or an individual's private space, where citizens might expect to exercise their free choice, without government interference.

Criticism of government intervention to protect individuals from harm is often heard with the pejorative term 'nanny state', which implies too much interference in the lives of individuals, limiting their freedom and choice. Baggott (2011) describes two contrasting political positions on the involvement of government in health matters: liberal-individualistic, which seeks to promote individual liberty and choice, free from government intrusion; and collectivist, which sees a role for the state in protecting communities through guidance, legislation, and taxation.

Critics of the liberal-individualistic approach argue that government intervention is necessary because people's choices are constrained by the social determinants which are not equally distributed: for example, poverty, poor housing, and stigma and discrimination. Legislation is also needed to protect vulnerable individuals, for example, in the case of domestic violence and child abuse.

To illustrate, Caraher and colleagues (2014) argue that the government can play an important role in tackling obesity by regulating the food industry. The authors argue that, as poorer people's food choices and access to healthy food are constrained by obesogenic environments (i.e. environments that contribute to obesity), they are more likely to be exposed to unhealthy choices. Moreover, unhealthy food is often cheaper than healthy food, and given the preponderance of fast-food outlets, available 24 hours a day, there is an increasing availability of unhealthy food. Intervention therefore needs to be levelled at industry, not only individuals. Fizzy drinks are a prime example, and in 2018 the Soft Drinks Industry Levy was introduced to reduce the level of sugar in soft drinks (HM Treasury, 2015). However this arrangement was largely voluntary, which, Caraher and Perry (2017) argue, was ineffective, suggesting 'harder regulation' of the industry is required. A recent systematic review of the literature also supported the need for tougher regulation, with the findings that food environments undermine initiatives for individuals to manage their weight, which challenges ideas, based on prejudice, that individuals are to blame for their obesity because of a lack of self-control (Neve and Isaacs, 2021). Indeed the government's policy paper on tackling obesity (DHSC, 2020) makes provision for legislation which restricts the promotion of unhealthy food, at checkouts and at the end of aisles, and replaces it with healthy options with the aim of changing people's spending and dietary habits.

Opponents of legislation would argue that people should be 'nudged' into changing their behaviour and making healthy food choices through positive reinforcement rather than enforcement: for example, placing healthy food at eye level in shops to encourage healthy choices (ESRC, 2021). Notwithstanding, the government has committed to restricting the promotion of unhealthy foods in 2022 as part of its strategy to tackle obesity, and will give local authorities powers to fine retailers who fall foul of the guidance to promote healthier choices (DHSC, 2021).

The Nuffield Council on Bioethics proposed a stewardship model illustrated by an 'intervention ladder' (see Figure 7.2) as a means of thinking about the acceptability of an intervention; these interventions range from providing information about how to keep healthy so people can make their own choices about how to manage their health, to the introduction of legislation to reduce fat and sugar content in food (i.e. eliminate choice). The Council argues that:

> *Any intervention should be proportionate to the effect that it is intended to achieve, and should be supported by evidence (or, in the absence of robust evidence, should be accompanied by an evidence-gathering programme). Interventions that are higher up the ladder are more intrusive and therefore require a stronger justification.*

(Nuffield Council on Bioethics, 2007)

| |
|---|
| Eliminate choice |
| Restrict choice |
| Guide choice by disincentives |
| Guide choice by incentives |
| Guide choice by changing the default policy |
| Enable choice |
| Provide information |
| Do nothing |

*Figure 7.2*   Nuffield ladder of intervention

© Nuffield Council on Bioethics (2007). The original version of this report *Public health: ethical issues* is available at www.nuffieldbioethics.org/publications/public-health

Early in the COVID-19 pandemic, governments everywhere used a range of public health measures to contain the virus. These included: a legal requirement to wear a face mask and social distancing; testing of individuals and tracing their contacts where test results proved positive and the isolation of infected individuals and their contacts; stay-at-home orders, including a requirement to work from home where possible; restrictions on the movement of the general population; and the banning or limiting of social gatherings.

As countries across the globe were hit by the outbreak, the disruption to normal life and the damage to people's livelihoods was unprecedented, with the poorest and most vulnerable populations hit the hardest. In some instances, these hardships were exacerbated by government interventions designed to protect individuals and communities and contain the spread of the virus (see examples provided earlier in the chapter).

Inaction (i.e. doing nothing) may also cause harm. A parliamentary report (House of Commons, 2021) into the government's handling of the crisis asserted that it was one of the worst public health failures in the UK. Its analysis of the government's response suggested that: the UK Government, having planned for an influenza pandemic, was not prepared for COVID-19 and formulated a response based on an outdated flu model. The government was late to lock down the country, believing that people would not accept the stay-at-home order. In general, the implementation of measures to curb the virus (social distancing, wearing of masks) was 'incremental and slow', which allowed the virus to spread. The government appeared to abandon traditional public health measures of testing the population to find those infected with the virus, and their contacts, to ensure they were isolated, due to a lack of testing capacity. The report concluded that the loss of life experienced in the first wave of the pandemic could have been prevented. Conversely, the UK vaccination programme has been heralded as one of the more effective responses of the government to the pandemic across Europe.

## Health Protection: should vaccination be mandatory?

Although there is an increasing body of evidence to support the protective effects of COVID-19 vaccination, there is opposition, and many citizens across the globe refused the vaccine or demonstrated vaccine hesitancy in the earlier vaccination programmes. Governments used a range of measures to encourage vaccination, including legislation: for example, Austria became the first country to make COVID-19 vaccination mandatory for all its citizens by February 2022, followed by Italy. Greece introduced mandatory vaccination, selectively, for those over 60, who faced fines for non-compliance (Chadwick, 2022). Many countries introduced legislation to make vaccination mandatory for health and social care workers and other key workers. Governments also used a range of incentives and disincentives. For example, in Germany, people were required to have proof of vaccination to access indoor arenas and were, therefore, effectively excluded from participating in many aspects of public life without vaccination. Some countries offered financial incentives to encourage vaccination. Many employers, concerned about the impact of workforce absence due to COVID-19, also required their employees to be vaccinated.

Mandatory vaccination is not unusual for childhood immunisation: for example, measles, mumps, and rubella (see the article by Marks and Vanderslott, 2021 for an interactive map of global childhood immunisation policies). There are examples of countries where vaccines are recommended (e.g. UK), mandatory (e.g. France), or mandated for children for school entry (e.g. Germany, the US).

Governments have justified vaccine mandates to protect the population, arguing that the collective good, and the need to protect vulnerable individuals, should take precedence over the right to individual liberty and freedom of choice. This was the case with the smallpox vaccination in the UK, which was mandatory until 1948.

Activity 7.4 requires you to reflect on your personal feelings about policies on mandatory vaccination for COVID-19 and other infectious diseases, including childhood immunisation.

## Activity 7.4   Reflection

Reflect on your personal views about the COVID-19 vaccine. Why do you think people are vaccine-hesitant? Should the vaccine be mandatory for health and social care staff and other key workers (for example, teachers and transport workers)? How far should the government intervene to protect individuals and communities by making COVID-19 vaccines, or childhood vaccination, mandatory? What different approaches could the government take to ensure higher take-up of the vaccine? Reflect on your views in relation to the Nuffield ladder of intervention (Figure 7.2) and the article by Marks and Vanderslott (2021).

*As the answers are based on your own reflections, there is no outline answer at the end of the chapter.*

# Health policy and diverse communities

The importance of the need for good health policy in tackling health inequalities is aptly described by the Commission on Social Determinants of Health:

> *[The] toxic combination of bad policies, economics, and politics is, in large measure, responsible for the fact that a majority of people in the world do not enjoy the good health that is biologically possible.*

> (WHO, 2008a, p26)

The above quote would appear to support a strong role for governments in improving health, and preventing ill health, through appropriate economic and political systems and policies that address inequalities.

Politics can be defined as *the process of influencing the allocation of scarce resources* (Chaffee et al., 2012, p5). McCullough (2014) quotes Shrock (1977), who argues that nurses should develop political awareness *to understand and analyse the socio-economic and political background to the services of which they are part, as a potentially powerful group of health care workers.*

Health policy:

> *refers to decisions, plans, and actions that are undertaken to achieve specific health care goals within a society. An explicit health policy can achieve several things: it defines a vision*

*for the future which in turn helps to establish targets and points of reference for the short and medium term. It outlines priorities and the expected roles of different groups and it builds consensus and informs people.*

(WHO, n.d.)

Governments introduce policies to address specific problems, and policies change over time due to political, social, economic, and cultural developments. Solutions to the problems the policy is trying to address also change over time. Abuse in older people, for example, is increasingly recognised as an issue, perhaps because of people living longer, as well as high-profile cases of abuse of trust by carers and changing attitudes towards older people. Policy does not exist in a vacuum, however, and an understanding of the drivers of policy and the political and economic landscape in which nurses are required to implement policy, as part of their practice, is an important aspect of public health. Table 7.1 outlines some policies influencing nursing practice in England.

| | |
|---|---|
| Our Vision for the Women's Health Strategy for England (Department of Health and Social Care, 2021) | Sets out the government's vision, based on a life course approach, to improve experiences of healthcare services and health outcomes for women and girls, and to reduce disparities in women's health. |
| Towards Zero: the HIV Action Plan for England – 2022 to 2025 (Department of Health and Social Care, 2021) | Outlines the actions the government will take to prevent people from getting HIV, ensure those who get HIV are diagnosed promptly, prevent onward transmission from those with diagnosed infection, and deliver interventions which improve the health and quality of life of people with HIV and reduce stigma. |
| From Harm to Hope: A 10-year plan to cut crime and save lives (Cross Departmental, 2021) | Sets out the government's plan to break drug supply chains, deliver a world-class treatment and recovery system, and achieve a generational shift in demand for drugs. |
| National Disability Strategy (Disability Unit and Equality Hub, 2021) | Outlines the government's vision to transform the everyday lives of disabled people by removing barriers and improving outcomes and opportunities for disabled people. |
| Tuberculosis (TB): Action plan for England, 2021 – 2026 (UK Health Security Agency, 2021) | Commits to improving the prevention, detection, and control of TB in England. |

*Table 7.1* Examples of policies guiding public health practice

# The drivers of contemporary policy

The factors that drive the need for policy may include:

- evidence of health needs (increases in rates of obesity, smoking, dementia, falls in older people, poor uptake of immunisation, etc.);
- changing societal attitudes and public opinion (e.g. concerns about violence, child health, and the need to protect vulnerable groups, and concerns about poverty and the impact on children's health and development);

- pressure groups demanding change and influencing policy, including healthcare professionals, the public, parents, professional bodies, trade unions, and voluntary organisations;
- economic costs of disease or welfare (costs to the government for treating diseases and the austerity agenda);
- recognition that current practice/service delivery is not fit for purpose and that change needs to be implemented (e.g. the Francis Report (Department of Health, 2013) into the failings of the Mid-Staffordshire NHS Foundation Trust, which recommended the need to develop standards of care; and the Morecambe Bay Investigation into the deaths of mothers and babies in 2013);
- evidence reviews (e.g. the Marmot Review on health inequalities); and
- ideology informed by the political positions of different governments (the referendum on leaving the European Union ('Brexit') was not based on evidence, but political ideas).

## Influencing policy and decision-making to change health systems and tackle inequalities

Action to bring about change in policies addressing poverty and inequality is a matter of social justice because some groups experience poorer health outcomes than others and are more adversely affected by policies. There is some evidence to suggest that women, minorities, and disabled people were worst hit by the impact of austerity measures implemented by the Conservative–Liberal Democrat Coalition Government (2010–2015), as were more deprived local authorities (Hastings et al., 2017). In this chapter, we have discussed how diverse communities were negatively impacted by policies which aimed to protect the wider population. Moreover, as nurses and midwives act as advocates for their clients/patients, they need to understand how to influence policy to protect vulnerable communities.

The health policy-making process consists of three stages: policy formulation, policy implementation, and policy reformation. It has been suggested that nurses and midwives do not engage with the policy process due to a perceived lack of *time and resources, lack of status and decision-making power and a possible lack of politicisation of nurses* (Gleeson et al., 2015, p40). However, there are different approaches that nurses and midwives can use to influence policy, including: through membership of a trade union (e.g. UNITE) or professional organisation such as the RCN, by contributing to government, national or local, consultation documents (e.g. on proposed changes to the NHS, legislation regulating sugar and salt content in food, regulation of healthcare professions), by writing to their MP or local councillor about an issue; and, by voting in the general and local elections. We provide an activity that would allow you to advocate on behalf of communities by writing to your MP (see Activity 7.5).

# Leadership: influencing policy

## Action to address the wider determinants of health: loneliness and social isolation

Social isolation and loneliness are serious but often unrecognised public health risks that affect a substantial proportion of the population. The term social isolation refers to the lack of social contacts and having few people to interact with regularly, while loneliness is the distressing feeling of being alone or separated. Social isolation and loneliness have been linked with an increased risk of premature death, a risk that may be similar to smoking, alcohol misuse, obesity, and physical inactivity. While social isolation and loneliness can affect anyone, high levels are reported by older people, care home residents, informal carers (i.e. family caregivers), and people with learning disabilities.

People with learning disabilities are up to seven times more likely to feel lonely than other people (MENCAP, 2020) and have fewer opportunities to participate in social and leisure activities than the general population. They also often feel unwanted in mainstream social settings and might need support to help communicate, meet, and interact with peers and develop long-term friendships.

Both austerity policies and the pandemic have increased the risk of social isolation and loneliness among people with learning disabilities. In terms of austerity, the accounts of people with learning disabilities describe how cuts to services led to them losing opportunities for meeting others, including becoming housebound and separated from their peers (Malli et al., 2018). The impact of COVID-19 was also difficult for many, due to the closure of day services, loss of routine, and limits on seeing people living in other households. Tackling the harms caused by austerity and the pandemic and creating a socially connected future for people with learning disabilities requires determination, innovation, and leadership.

In the field of public health, leadership relates to the ability of an individual to influence, motivate, and enable others to contribute toward the effectiveness and success of their community and/or the organisation in which they work (Public Health Agency of Canada, 2016). During the Coronavirus pandemic, we saw examples of leadership from government advisors, such as the Chief Medical Officer for England, Professor Chris Whitty, whose role was to advise the government on the science underpinning the effectiveness of measures required to slow the spread of transmission of the virus. Other healthcare practitioners, such as Dr Becks Fisher, a GP, set up a Health Foundation Research Partnership to track the experiences of GPs, practice nurses, and practice managers as they responded to the pandemic. We also saw examples of leadership from ordinary citizens, including those residents who signed up with their local authorities as COVID-19 Health Champions and who shared evidence-based health messages and guidance with their friends, families, and communities. Another prominent leader in the field of public health and community well-being was Marcus

Rashford, a professional footballer with Manchester United, who campaigned to tackle child hunger and lobbied the government to provide free school meals in England during the summer holidays. His campaigning prompted a major change in government policy. He was subsequently recognised in the Queen's Birthday Honours list and awarded an MBE.

Activity 7.5 invites you to demonstrate your leadership capabilities in order to influence policy, motivate, and enable others to reduce social isolation and loneliness amongst people with learning disabilities.

## Activity 7.5   Communication

We have seen that people with learning disabilities are disproportionately affected by social isolation and loneliness. While the National Disability Strategy outlined the government's vision to transform the everyday lives of disabled people by removing barriers and improving outcomes and opportunities for disabled people, disabled people's organisations have criticised the policy for being insubstantial and lacking the concrete measures needed to tackle the growing poverty, exclusion, and discrimination disabled people face (Pring, 2021). These groups are calling for the strategy to be reviewed and campaigning for radical plans with timescales, and financial investment to make change a reality. What would you do to support their campaign, with particular reference to loneliness and social isolation?

*An outline answer is provided at the end of the chapter.*

## Chapter summary

We began the chapter with an overview of epidemiology, the changing patterns of disease and the public health measures designed to tackle these health challenges. We have demonstrated how resurgent diseases, for example, tuberculosis, a significant health threat in the nineteenth and early twentieth centuries in the UK, now targets the most deprived communities and requires continuous monitoring and attention given the significant global burden and risk of co-infection for those with HIV-AIDS. An understanding of epidemiology is important to monitor changing patterns of disease, and to anticipate future trends, in order to plan health and social care, and associated interventions which need to be tailored to meet the specific needs of diverse communities.

We discussed the specific health needs of diverse communities that often experience worse health, and health outcomes, compared to the general population. Although people are living longer, they are more likely to be living with a preventable disabling condition (e.g. T2D) which can impact their health and quality of life. We have argued that inequalities in health cannot be explained by biology or genetics alone, but also by social determinants (i.e. the conditions in which people are born, live, grow, work, and age). Tackling the social determinants of health inequalities will have implications for nursing practice and the wider NHS and social care services.

Health inequalities were particularly marked during the earlier phase of the COVID-19 pandemic, where we witnessed the unequal impact on diverse communities, including those experiencing deprivation, attributed to: 'differential exposure', 'differential vulnerability', and differential access to resources and measures to mitigate risk (Katikireddi et al., 2021). We also highlighted how diverse communities were adversely affected by generic pandemic prevention measures designed to protect the public. This demonstrates an important role for nurses and midwives in influencing policy, and advocating for the communities they serve, to ensure they are not disadvantaged by new policies, or changes in policy, or policies that appear to work well for the general population but may significantly disadvantage some communities.

Readers will be struck by the significance of the role of vaccination programmes in the eradication of disease, both historically, in preventing childhood illness, and in the present, and the crucial role the vaccination programme has played in relation to COVID-19. Vaccine hesitancy, although not a new concept, presents a significant barrier to the success of the COVID-19 vaccination programme and we discussed a range of measures governments have used to maximise the uptake of vaccines. Governments have an important role to play in protecting the health of the public, including the funding of the NHS through taxation. How much governments are willing to intervene in the lives of citizens, however, is highly political and this has been the case in relation to specific measures to curb the spread of COVID-19 (for example, the lack of a clear and consistent approach to the wearing of face masks during different phases of the pandemic).

However, given the differential exposure, vulnerabilities, and risks that diverse communities already experience suggests a non-interventionist stance could exacerbate inequalities, as not everyone has access to resources that enable healthy choices. Nurses and midwives will have to exercise skill and judgement in supporting people to make the best choices they can within the constraints and vulnerabilities they face. The importance of a public health preventative approach in relation to T2D, for example, is ever-pressing given that diabetes is one of the leading causes of lower foot amputation, which can be avoided through appropriate foot care and better management of diabetes. The proposed restrictions on the promotion of unhealthy food in retail stores to tackle obesity demonstrate that the government does recognise the value of intervention, through legislation, to promote healthier food choices (DHSC, 2020, 2021); however, some of the measures outlined in the obesity strategy have been deferred until 2023, and it remains to be seen whether they will be implemented at all.

We have discussed the role of evidence-informing policies in tackling inequalities (e.g. the role of epidemiology underpinning the Marmot Review) and provided examples of policies that may exacerbate inequalities, suggesting that nurses and midwives need to be able to exercise political awareness in order to influence policy-making, tackle inequalities, and improve nursing care. Nurses and midwives who have a better understanding of the health needs of diverse communities will also be able to oppose policies and legislation that discriminate against, and further disadvantage, particular sections of the community by registering their concerns with policy and lawmakers.

# Activities: brief outline answers

## Activity 7.5   Leadership (p150)

One of the ways that Marcus Rashford brought about change in relation to child hunger was by writing a letter to his MP. Many people write to their MPs every year. MPs depend on their constituents to educate them about the issues that are important to them. One way to demonstrate leadership would be to write to your MP.

A standard pattern to use when writing a letter to a decision-maker, such as a councillor or MP, is the EPIC format (see the useful websites section at the end of the chapter). EPIC stands for:

- *Engage:* Say something that is attention-grabbing. For example, outline the findings from a listening exercise with people with learning disabilities about their experiences of social isolation and loneliness during the pandemic.

- *Problem:* Explain the precise nature of the problem. For example, describe the health and social inequalities experienced by people with learning disabilities, and the link between loneliness and poor health outcomes.

- *Inform:* Inform the MP of what a potential solution to the problem might be. For example, SENSE, a charity that champions the rights of disabled people, has called for action on:

  o Accessibility for disabled people to be integrated into all programmes aiming to tackle loneliness

  o Government programmes to provide appropriate funding for social care, and for local authorities to deliver improved, more accessible services that tackle loneliness, as well as opportunities that allow disabled people to explore and interact with others in their community

  o A more accessible society, with attention to transport, public buildings and homes, so that disabled people can access social opportunities

- *Call to action:* Explain exactly what the MP can do to help. For example, you could ask the MP to raise a question in the House of Commons to highlight the problem, which could lead to the National Disability Strategy being reviewed and more concrete measures being put in place to create a socially connected future for people with learning disabilities.

You can find a copy of the letter Marcus Rashford sent to his MP at: https://greenbank-primary.co.uk/wp-content/uploads/2020/07/marcus-rashford-letter-to-parliament.pdf.

# Further Reading

**The Kings Fund** (2022) What are health inequalities? Available at: **www.kingsfund.org.uk/publications/what-are-health-inequalities** (accessed 10 November 2022).

# Useful websites

The UCL Institute of Health Equity aims to inform evidence-based policies based on research, and support approaches to health equity:

**www.instituteofhealthequity.org/about-us/the-institute-of-health-equity**

They work for you: use this website to identify your local MP:

**www.theyworkforyou.com**

How to write to your MP: additional guidance on how to write to your MP/decision-maker, using the EPIC framework:

**https://resultscanada.ca/wp-content/uploads/how-to-write-to-your-MP.pdf**

Pathway: Healthcare for Homeless People:

**www.pathway.org.uk/faculty**

Use this website to find out about inclusion health for excluded groups, such as vulnerable migrants, sex workers, Gypsies, and Travellers.

SENSE: Find out about the needs of deaf/blind people and those with complex disabilities:

**www.sense.org.uk**

# Chapter 8  Mental distress and cultural diversity

*Nicky Lambert and Beverley Brathwaite*

## NMC Future Nurse: Standards of Proficiency for Registered Nurses

This chapter will address the following platforms and proficiencies:

**Platform 1: Being an accountable professional**

1.14  provide and promote non-discriminatory, person-centred, and sensitive care at all times, reflecting on people's values and beliefs, diverse backgrounds, cultural characteristics, language requirements, needs and preferences, taking account of any need for adjustments.

**Platform 2: Promoting health and preventing ill health**

2.2  demonstrate knowledge of epidemiology, demography, genomics and the wider determinants of health, illness, and well-being and apply this to an understanding of global patterns of health and well-being outcomes.

2.3  understand the factors that may lead to inequalities in health outcomes.

## Chapter aims

After reading this chapter, you will be able to:

- explore the factors that impact on the well-being of people with mental health issues who are from minority backgrounds;
- describe ethical practice when working with people with mental health issues; and
- identify your key responsibilities in ensuring best practice when working with people with mental health issues.

# Introduction

- In 1914, a psychiatrist at the Georgia State Sanatorium, Dr EM Green, published research finding a higher rate of psychosis in African Americans than in their white counterparts; 100 years later, these findings are still resonating in the UK.
- Kirkbride et al. (2008) and Qassem et al. (2015) both identified that people from Black and Brown (B&B) communities are more likely to experience psychosis than the white majority population, and McManus et al. (2009) found that 3.1 per cent of African Caribbean men have a risk of psychosis, compared with 0.2 per cent of white men.
- What is striking about this obvious disparity in the UK is that rates of psychosis in the Caribbean and Africa are not as elevated. This suggests that rather than mental health issues being an inbuilt, genetic hazard for people from B&B backgrounds, there are aspects of living as a minority community that put some people at higher risk of mental distress (van Os, 2012).
- There are multiple barriers to B&B men expressing psychological distress and racial trauma is one of them in the UK. (Gsbertha, 2023).

This chapter begins with the above statistics, which show differences in the well-being of people from B&B backgrounds that are both striking and unfair. The issues around mental health (MH) and diversity, particularly cultural diversity, are long-standing and emotive. There should be a parity of esteem between physical and mental health. This means that both are equally as important to a person's total wellbeing and should be addressed as such when caring for patients (Coupland, 2023). It is essential to have a level of understanding of these issues in order to give compassionate and effective care. This chapter helps you to explore some of the issues around cultural diversity that can affect people's MH. It also has practical suggestions for working ethically and effectively with all the people in your community.

First, we introduce the idea that language shapes the way that we think, talk, and act, and that this in turn has real-world implications for people's health. We then explore the health issues that affect those from minority cultures and their experience of discrimination in health services. We will go on to explore how MH services can be more accessible and effective in giving care to people from minority backgrounds. The chapter ends with suggestions on how we can give better care as individuals and members of the health service.

The language surrounding diversity can be complicated, and this has been looked at in Chapters 1 and 2 of this book. It is important to remember that an individual's identity or *sense of self* is often more complex than definitions allow and that everyone receiving services is an individual who should receive personalised care.

Another idea that you will see in discussions about culture is the *minority population*. The social majority are those who dominate positions of power in society; minority populations are those who do not. A person's minority status might be visible due to religious or cultural dress, or unseen in a condition such as autism. It might be permanent in the form of an individual's ethnicity or temporary such as a mental health issue. It can even be a combination of these, such as a Black Muslim woman with autism.

A minority population is not defined by numbers, but by proximity and access to social power (e.g. women make up just over half of the UK population but are considered a minority group because of the dominance of men in positions of authority and the social impacts which that entails).

Rethinking Mental Illness (2021, pp1–2) notes that if you are from a Black, Asian, or Minority Ethnic (BAME) background, you may experience different rates of mental illness than the white population. Fear, stigma, and lack of culturally sensitive treatment can act as barriers to accessing mental healthcare. More white people receive treatment for MH issues than people from B&B backgrounds and they have better outcomes. There are also variances in this picture between different minority groups and gender compared to white people:

- Black women are more likely to experience a common mental illness such as anxiety disorder or depression
- Older South Asian women are an at-risk group for suicide
- Black men are more likely to experience psychosis
- Black people are four times more likely to be detained under the Mental Health Act.

These findings raise concerns about social justice, racism, prejudice, and stigma, as well as diagnosis, treatment, and the experience of care in mental health services. It is useful to examine the language commonly used in policy and research to understand and address these issues and to provide context for them.

You might wonder why a consideration of language is important to your ability to give compassionate and effective care, but healthcare is embedded in social systems and the health of individuals is shaped directly by the world they experience. The terms BAME/BME have been constantly contested by social scientists for some time, but now the government even acknowledges how unuseful they have become (Race Disparity Unit, 2022). Also, with the publication of the Commission on Race and Ethnic Disparity Report (CRED, 2021) and *COVID-19: Understanding the Impact on BAME Communities* (PHE, 2020b) highlighting the impact of COVID-19 on minoritised groups, they have figured out that there is a need to look at social groups specifically, such as Black African or Asian. Other marginalised experiences within minority communities include those of Irish, Gypsy, Roma, and Traveller (GRT) peoples, who are sometimes called 'unseen minorities', because while experiencing significant disadvantages in terms of their health, they are not always considered in discussions of BAME/BME concerns. Hence another reason why we use the term B&B within this edition of the book.

Understanding the impact of diversity and the language used around it is central to being a professional working within the Nursing and Midwifery Council Code (NMC, 2018b), in order to uphold people's dignity, champion their rights, and challenge discrimination. Good MH care is dependent on an individual's recovery journey and can be dependent on active social engagement and a positive sense of self. If someone is excluded because of racism or stigma towards their identity, their return to health is likely to be affected. It is also important to appreciate that culture, heritage, language, and religion shape an individual's experience of their own mental health. These factors can also affect the way their friends and family respond to them if they need help, particularly as mental illness can be a source of shame and fear in many cultures (Sangar and Howe, 2021).

With the changing demographics of minoritised communities (especially in cities), local health services continue to use BAME but tend to acknowledge it is problematic and its limitations (MH, UK, n.d.). In order to address specific needs, benchmark quality, and commission appropriate services, we need ways to describe prevalence, incidence, and outcomes for non-white communities, so for the moment terminology such as BAME remains in use.

Discrimination in society and within services has been long recognised. The Department of Health's Delivering Race Equality in Mental Health Care Plan (2005) identified 12 characteristics that it was hoped would improve mental healthcare for all by 2010. Areas of action include:

* reducing fear of services in B&B communities;
* encouraging greater levels of participation by minoritised communities in co-producing services, policy, and professional education;
* improving service user satisfaction and recovery rates;
* reducing the disproportionate numbers of people from B&B communities being admitted under the Mental Health Act;
* improving minoritised access to talking therapies;
* ensuring that prescriptions of medication were appropriate and effective;
* reducing the levels of violence occurring in mental health services. This focused on reducing the practices of restraining and secluding people who became aggressive while mentally distressed and preventing injury or deaths where restraint proved unavoidable.

These issues continue and the COVID-19 pandemic has only exacerbated some of these (Nazroo et al., 2020; Jaspal and Lopes, 2021). Having explored some of these ideas, we will now look at some of the reasons this might be the case in Activity 8.1.

## Activity 8.1 Critical thinking

So far, this chapter has established that people from minoritised communities often have a poorer experience than other sectors of society when it comes to accessing and receiving mental healthcare in the UK. It is a complicated picture, but from your own observations and what you have read, note down some of the reasons that you think might be the cause.

*Because these are your own ideas, there is no outline answer provided. However, look at the Rethink Mental Illness Fact Sheet (2021) (available at: www.rethink.org/advice-and-information/living-with-mental-illness/wellbeing-physical-health/black-asian-and-minority-ethnic-mental-health/) to give you some evidence-based reasons.*

Having looked at your own ideas on why minoritised communities may have poorer mental health experiences in Activity 8.1, we will now review some of the theories advanced by others. Consider how they agree with your own ideas, as well as where they differ.

# Social inequality

Minoritised communities experience higher levels of poverty, increased unemployment, and poorer living conditions than the general population and these factors are linked to poorer health outcomes (Marmot et al., 2020b). Public awareness and open discussions around mental health are thankfully growing. The first project of the Office for Health Improvement and Disparities (OHID), New Every Mind Matters campaign to improve people's mental health (GOV.UK, 2021), launched during the pandemic is an example of campaigns to improve the MH of the population. Like all public health activities, they can be hard to measure in terms of proven outcomes and are often hindered rather than helped by the political process, economic pressures, and short-termism, which during the COVID-19 pandemic, are all even more of an issue.

# Racism and institutionalised racism

> *Fatal incidents involving Black patients speak to the most glaring cases of institutional racism in British mental health settings. These tragedies are translated into inquiries – usually only produced following extraordinary efforts from the families of victims.*
>
> (Younis, 2021, p1833)

Empathy enables us to make the connection between abuse and distress. It seems obvious that facing racism and discrimination could diminish an individual's resilience, as well as that of their community, leading to increased levels of mental distress (Bamford et al., 2021). However, institutionalised racism can prove more challenging to think about. Most people who enter health and social care do so to provide services in a compassionate and respectful way, so it can be hard to appreciate that as a whole, the system can unintentionally produce outcomes that may harm individuals. For example, care pathways designed without stakeholder input, and which are monitored by quality measures that ignore the experience, satisfaction, and recovery rates of minority communities, may result in poor outcomes that are overlooked.

Black people with African Caribbean heritage are more likely than any other group to be diagnosed and admitted to hospital with psychosis (Brown, 2022). It has been suggested that these higher rates are caused by social and economic disadvantages (Nazroo et al., 2020) or health professionals making negative assumptions about people, particularly young Black men, and pathologising cultural differences (Younis, 2021). Health provision reflects the society of its time, and there is a disturbing history of problematic power relations within MH care, shaping life chances, interpersonal interactions, and encounters with institutions. Race/ethnicity has real effects and is a result of the historically and politically shaped meanings of racism (Nazroo et al., 2020).

Younis (2021) identifies that Black men have become increasingly linked to psychosis and UK findings have reported this consistently for more than 60 years (Nazroo et al., 2020). Relating Black men particularly to psychotic symptoms such as 'hostility' and 'aggression' became part of the diagnostic criteria for schizophrenia in the *Diagnostic and Statistical Manual of Mental Disorders* (which defines and classifies mental illnesses for the American Psychiatric Association). An advertisement for an anti-psychotic medication called Haldol from the Archives of General Psychiatry demonstrated at best a fearful and controlling attitude towards Black masculinity (Anakwenze, 2020). This helped to build on and reinforce institutional racism in the UK as well as in America. As a practice note, do not forget that most countries use the *International Statistical Classification of Diseases and Related Health Problems* (ICD-10) from the World Health Organization (WHO) for diagnostic criteria, and that there are differences between the two.

We have been exploring the impact of racism on MH; however, stigma can be more subtle in practice. Look at Activity 10.2 and consider how you might respond to it.

## Activity 8.2   Critical reflection

The misuse of institutional and professional power has always been with us in society, and one of the most interesting but dangerous aspects of working in mental health is that it sometimes gives you the authority to define what is 'normal' or acceptable and what is not. In order to practise compassionately and ethically, you need to consider how you think about people who are different to you and be reflective about the results of your actions as well as your intentions. How might you handle the following situation?

> *You hear a colleague saying that a young man from an African background with depression and anxiety isn't suitable for a referral to CBT or talking therapies because he probably couldn't 'think it through as he's more physical'.*

Write down your response to this situation.

*There are outline answers at the end of the chapter that you may find helpful.*

Activity 8.2 is intended to help you to think about ways to manage the power and responsibility that can accompany the privilege of working with people who may be vulnerable due to mental distress. It can be hard sometimes to appreciate the difference between our professional judgement and personal beliefs and prejudices. An example of this occurred when, in 1851, an American, Dr Samuel Cartwright, came across a behaviour that he could not rationally explain and believed that he had discovered a new mental illness. He presented his findings to acclaim in the southern states, suggesting that this 'new' mental illness, drapetomania, was what caused Black slaves to run away from captivity (White, 2002).

It seems obvious to us today that an individual attempting to escape slavery is not ill; Cartwright's ideas were met with derision in the North and have never been recognised as part of established diagnoses. I have included them to demonstrate that we can all be blind to our own prejudice and have an obligation to be cautious because our professional judgements can have such serious consequences for other people. Indeed, research by Holland and Ousey (2011) and Weerasinghe (2012) found that even today, just having an accent and wearing clothing that signifies a B&B identity can make people vulnerable to discrimination.

Another perspective on this issue came from the *Aetiology and Ethnicity in Schizophrenia and Other Psychoses* study – AESOP for short (Morgan et al., 2006). It suggested the hypothesis that experience of urban poverty is what raises the risk of mental distress, not B&B identity, and that higher numbers of socially excluded B&B communities in urban areas may explain their higher rates of diagnosis. Arguably, this is a rather circular argument, as structural inequalities based on racial discrimination are one of the things confining minority populations to poor housing and limited incomes in the first place.

# Fear of mental health services

Most people are treated for mental distress in primary care, and while it is fair to say few people who are referred on to specialist services are enthusiastic about coming into contact with MH professionals, their trajectory is very different to the 40 per cent of people from B&B communities referred through the criminal justice system (Kane, 2014). Certainly, B&B communities are over-represented within the criminal justice system, which may account for some of this percentage; however, there are likely to be several other factors.

It may be that B&B communities are less aware of what help is available (Fernando and Keating, 2009) and struggle to access services if they are not confident English speakers or aware of procedures. Equally, it may well be that they avoid statutory services because of poor previous experiences. It is likely that people avoid services that are not thought to be culturally sensitive or that may bring stigma to individuals and their families (Mereish et al., 2012). It may also be that some communities feel that caregiving is a family responsibility (Cooper et al., 2013), and so they wait until a health issue has become unmanageable in the community (Kane, 2014). Indeed, Morgan et al. (2006) found that not only do some carers from some B&B communities delay accessing health services, but when they are forced by necessity to seek statutory help, they call the police before a doctor.

# The culture of mental health services

We have focused thus far on cultural differences in minority populations, but all groups have beliefs, traditions, and attitudes that bind them together. Fernando (2003, 2010) is a key thinker in exploring ideas of cultural dissonance (i.e. the 'culture clash' that can occur between psychiatry and people from non-Western backgrounds).

Psychiatric concepts come from a Western, post-Enlightenment tradition. They are still largely biomedical in focus and contain ideas of 'illness' and 'normality' that may not resonate with B&B communities, who may have a more holistic approach or belief in supernatural causations. Health professionals are usually from a background that has certain privileges, such as access to higher education, status, and regular income. This can differentiate them from the people they often end up caring for. There is also an assumption of 'objectivity' in professional identity and the unspoken assumption that diagnosis is a scientific process. This may lead health professionals to over-inflate their confidence in their own judgement rather than encourage them to pause to ask questions and clarify misunderstandings.

MH services evolved out of the asylum system, where people who might be a risk to themselves or others were removed from society. The assumed link between 'madness' and danger can result in pressure on professionals to be made responsible for public safety. This can result in professionals who may be risk-averse and who may not always appreciate that sadness, fear, and anger can look very different across cultural boundaries.

# Politics before and during the COVID-19 pandemic

One of the most challenging aspects of understanding MH issues and cultural diversity is what Nutbeam (2004) called *analysis paralysis*. This occurs where evidence of a problem grows but there is no organised policy implementation to address it. One reason for this is that the current political trajectory in health provision is a neoliberal one. An example of this is that the research linking deprivation to poorer health outcomes – an issue that is key to the well-being of minoritised communities – has not been translated into meaningful action.

The MH policy paper *No Health without Mental Health* (Department of Health, 2011) suggests that 'resilience' can protect against MH difficulties. Larsson (2013) notes that the social impacts of exclusion and deprivation on the health of individuals and their communities are replaced by vague advice that individuals should be 'mentally tough'. To put this suggestion into perspective, imagine the reaction to a physical health policy that suggested people at specific risk of ill health could 'will' physical illness away.

Knapp (2012) provides an example of the inadequacy of the MH commissioning responses to this paper in the rollout of IAPT services (individual psychological interventions). The economic downturn increased social difficulties such as unemployment, and talking therapies, however well delivered, could not offer a practical remedy to these problems. Having counselling services in Job Centres can lead to vulnerable people being held personally responsible for issues caused by broader social problems. For example, in a recession, there are fewer jobs, and people discriminated against because of racism and stigmatised because they have mental health issues may find work harder to obtain. Therapy for these individuals does not change societal ills such as unemployment but may leave people feeling scapegoated if they struggle to find work.

When the lockdown came into effect the usual way of accessing MH services drastically changed and the daily routines that we all had were disrupted. As the pandemic went on the death rate increased and dealing with bereavement and grief in exceptional circumstances took place. Isolation across the board for the population became a bigger issue, which worsened the MH of already isolated older people and minoritised communities with ongoing MH issues (Diaz et al., 2021). The lack of preparedness of government policy when dealing with the pandemic has been reviewed and the effect this had on both physical and MH outcomes in relation to COVID-19 indicates reduced wellness in the population (Byrne et al., 2021). The lasting impact on the MH of the population will be felt for some time to come and, as we have seen, minoritised groups have borne the brunt of the mental distress caused by reduced access to services, poor experiences when dealing with MH services, having to access services in a different way, and lack of human contact (Bamford et al., 2021; Moore et al., 2021).

These factors can seem overwhelming and certainly much bigger than our individual scope of practice, but understanding them will put you in a position where you can respond to problems in care provision with professional integrity. Your choices not only support the recovery of people in mental distress; they shape the teams you work in. Whether you mean to or not, you act as a role model, and when people see your good practice, that impacts their actions. Policy writing and service commissioning can feel far removed from your everyday work, but policy is written by people – it doesn't just happen! So, it is important that you understand how to make informed decisions and put yourself forward to learn how to participate in this process and shape care for the better. The scenario below is designed to help you consider some of the big ideas we have looked at in a practice context.

## Scenario: working with linguistic diversity

Hibaq Yasin, a 58-year-old woman originally from Somalia, has been feeling dizzy when she stands up suddenly. She talks to her friend who had heart problems after similar symptoms and decides to visit her GP for advice. She hasn't used NHS services since her children were born. She had postnatal depression after the birth of her first child, and she says it was caused by being new in the country, as well as being lonely, with no family nearby. Her 15-year-old grandson accompanies her as she is very worried about her heart and gets anxious with people she doesn't know. Mrs Yasin can't remember some of the words when she describes her symptoms to the doctor, and her grandson helps her by translating her account of her room spinning when she sat up in bed.

The doctor looks confused, so she demonstrates feeling dizzy and fainting to show him. It is quite dramatic! The GP sees she has a history of mental health issues, so he asks her whether she has any unusual powers or hears voices in her head. Mrs Yasin is baffled but tries to be helpful. When the GP suggests she can see a mental health specialist, she is taken aback and very offended. She says she has never been to a 'mad doctor' and won't go now; she denies having used mental health services when the GP mentions her postnatal depression.

After some confusion, the situation is resolved when Mrs Yasin uses a colloquial expression to describe her dizziness, saying that the room was spinning around her head when she sat up; her grandson mistranslated and told the doctor that her grandmother thought she flew around her bedroom. The doctor asks Mrs Yasin if she thinks she can fly; she giggles and shakes her head. Eventually, Mrs Yasin remembers the word for dizzy and the appointment gets back on track.

The above scenario shows how easy it is for even a straightforward situation such as a consultation for suspected postural hypotension to become complicated when people are talking at cross purposes. Activity 8.3 gives you a chance to respond to the scenario and offer some solutions.

## Activity 8.3   Reflection

Critically reflect on the situation described in the above scenario. What factors contributed to the conversation becoming confused?

What could you do to give good care in a situation such as this?

*There are some suggested answers at the end of the chapter that you might find helpful.*

Activity 8.3 was designed to help you to apply the theories we have explored in the abstract to a practice situation. It was adapted and anonymised from real practice experiences, but unfortunately there have also been real cases that bring together a lot of the ideas we have encountered (NSC NHS Strategic Health Authority, 2003; Prins et al., 1993), as the case study below demonstrates.

## Case study: the death of David Bennett

On 30 October 1998, David 'Rocky' Bennett, a 38-year-old African Caribbean man, died after being restrained at a medium secure unit in Norfolk. While the unit had service users from different backgrounds, it was a predominantly culturally white staff group.

Mr Bennett came to the UK when he was 8 years old. He was a Rastafarian who enjoyed drumming; he was offered a traineeship by Chelsea Football Club in his late teens and had worked as a signwriter before being diagnosed with schizophrenia.

At about 10 p.m., an argument between Mr Bennett and another service user arose over the use of the phone. After a struggle, Mr Bennett hit the other service user, who responded with racial abuse. Staff tried to de-escalate the situation but decided to move one of the men overnight to another ward to defuse the situation. They decided to move Mr Bennett; however, he was aggrieved by this decision as, from his perspective, he had been racially abused and was now being moved as a punishment while the perpetrator was allowed to stay in his room. Mr Bennett became angry when informed that he would be staying overnight and punched a nurse three times, resulting in the restraint by staff that ultimately led to his death.

Mr Bennett was restrained face down on the floor with up to five nurses attempting to hold him. The injuries he sustained during this incident were consistent with excessive force. The staff tried to resuscitate him with oxygen, but by the time an ambulance arrived he had been unconscious for ten minutes. Shortly afterwards, he was pronounced dead.

### Findings

- The inquiry into the death of Mr Bennett found no evidence of deliberate misconduct, but the lead nurse was found to be negligent in *not following restraint protocol* to monitor consciousness and manage signs of distress. The restraint was mishandled by the nursing staff, with Mr Bennett's capacity to breathe restricted and the restraint continuing longer than was safe.
- There was *inadequate resuscitation* equipment in the ward, and a doctor, who might have been able to help, took more than an hour to arrive at the clinic.
- There were *irregularities in Mr Bennett's prescription* as he was getting heavy doses of three anti-psychotic drugs. This is poor practice. It was not thought to have been a significant influence on his death; it is, however, likely to have impacted the quality of his life.
- The report noted the *poor treatment of Mr Bennett's family*, who did not receive a timely apology or a timely, transparent account of the incident.
- No evidence of deliberate racism was suggested, and individuals were noted to have been kind. However, the report noted that Mr Bennett's *cultural, social, and religious needs had been overlooked* during his time at the clinic.

In 1993, Mr Bennett had written to the nursing director, pointing out:

> *As you know, there are over half a dozen Black boys in this clinic. I don't know if you have real-ised that there are no Africans on your staff at the moment. We feel there should be at least two Black persons in the medical or social work staff. For the obvious reasons of security and content-ment for all concerned please do your best to remedy this appalling situation.*

> (NSC NHS Strategic Health Authority, 2003, p9)

This case was pivotal in MH services changing their approach to cultural diversity, and it led to public debate and service reviews. Staff training and research have improved the management of violence and aggression, and while things are far from perfect, work practices have improved since this report was released. The Promotion of Safe and Therapeutic Services (PSTS) approaches that have been adopted across services and initiatives, such as the Safewards model (Bowers et al., 2015), encourage the use of verbal de-escalation and techniques to support people who are acutely disturbed with greater levels of compassion and safely. Racism and verbal harassment are formally part of risk assessments and are seen as triggers for staff to act. While debates around insti-tutional racism and poor responses to families when things go wrong remain highly charged, these subjects are regular topics for discussion and critique now.

As previously stated, minority communities are varied, and their health needs are not static; they can vary in response to life events across the life span. For example, recent immigrants and asylum seekers are likely to have been exposed to significant uncer-tainty and anxiety, personal losses, and forced migration. They are at higher risk of having depression, anxiety, and post-traumatic stress as a result of being culturally dis-oriented on reaching the UK, as well as being emotionally damaged by experiencing racism and a hostile political system (Jannesari et al., 2020).

At the other end of the life span are the experiences of older adults, with Tran et al. (2008) suggesting that older adults from Chinese communities may be underserved as they are less likely to recognise symptoms of mental distress as a health issue, and in systems that require 'self-report', they may be disadvantaged. Johl et al. (2016) found many of these same issues when looking at dementia within B&B communi-ties and GRT people report experiencing longer-term effects of MH issues (Hayanga et al., 2022). There is a disproportionally higher risk of dementia in B&B communities (Dodd et al., 2022). Working well with diverse populations is an area that will only grow in importance as at present the population is relatively young, but this will change, and the current approach to managing MH requires early identification and engagement with services.

The issues that we have considered in this chapter have all been big and complex – racism, identity, culture, and stigma – and trying to address them can feel overwhelming; however, there are lots of things that you can do to make the support that you give better.

## Activity 8.4    Decision-making

When you work with people across a range of backgrounds, consider your own practice. What decisions do you make that help people from diverse communities experience good care? Have a look at the list in the next section and think about skills you already have and consider ways to improve your practice. Remember to note the things you do well already, as well as the things you may need to read up on or do differently.

*As this answer is based on your own observation, there is no outline answer at the end of the chapter.*

# Best practice for working with people from minority communities in mental distress

As an individual practitioner, considering the following will help you to practise confidently when working with people from minority communities in mental distress.

## Your attitude

Providing care for people is a privilege, and to do that well you will need to know about the lives and experiences of people who are different from you. Push yourself to engage with films, books, and art that help you to see things from other people's perspectives.

Being culturally competent and anti-racist involves you being open-minded and working to inform yourself about the lives of those whom you are supporting. You should consider a person's background as well as their individuality to avoid pathologising personal and cultural preferences. Ensure that you do not make clinical decisions based on inaccurate stereotypes.

## Your knowledge

Make sure that you are aware of the ways that people from culturally diverse backgrounds might talk about or show mental distress. If a service user is described to you as paranoid, for example, consider that behaviour in light of social realities, and be someone that people are able to talk to about any form of stigma that they might experience.

Be prepared to tolerate some uncertainty when trying to understand other people's experiences and learn to cultivate humility with regard to the limits of your personal and professional understanding. Ask for help when you need it!

Be aware of the rights of service users and address any stigma or discrimination you are aware of. This might mean supporting an individual to complain, contacting an advocate, or speaking up on behalf of someone. Anyone can raise a concern if they feel the safety of patients, or the public is at risk (NMC, 2019). Your workplace will also have a policy, and you should contact your union if you have concerns as to how speaking up may be received.

# Professional approaches

*Personalisation* means that we adapt to the needs of the individual rather than assuming 'one size fits all'. It is a way of working with a *strengths-based model*, where care builds on people's autonomy, resilience, and abilities rather than making assumptions about what is best for someone from beliefs based on their diagnosis.

Care is given in a social context, and it is important that professionals provide *holistic care*. This means making sure that you look beyond the biomedical model and factor in the impact of disadvantage and unmet needs on someone's experience when you are caring for them.

As a service, we should be considering the following in order to better support people from minority communities in mental distress.

# Co-production

*Co-production* moves care provision on from tokenistic service user involvement to bringing stakeholder expertise into the core of decision-making and agenda-setting of the service. This can include anything from supporting service users to evaluate the services they use, to capacity-building by including peer mentors as part of the workforce. Statutory services can also help provide the infrastructure to develop *communities of interest*. They are well-placed to forge links with a range of specialist and community-based organisations. Many voluntary organisations provide flexible and tailored services that support the mental and physical health of B&B communities; however, funding is rarely secure for long, which can undermine their efforts. A *community of interest* between statutory and voluntary partners can share intelligence, work together to provide an evidence base for best practice, work as advocates, and act as a reference point.

# Commissioning and research

We can work with service users and researchers to commission an *evidence base* for best practice in supporting the MH of minority communities. Commissioning agreements should be formulated to ensure that services collect routine data on outcomes for varied minoritised communities so that we can benchmark services to identify good practice to share.

Given the historically poor relationship between MH services and minority communities, public mental health initiatives could be designed to reach this community, tackling the stigma around mental distress and signposting people towards help. The inequalities that exist within minoritised populations and MH care cannot be explained by a *variable disease burden model*, and we need a better understanding of the experience and outcomes of MH treatment among B&B groups. We would benefit from a clear research and action plan. Indeed, in light of the harm caused by stigma and discrimination more generally, there is also a case to suggest that racism itself should be treated as a public health issue because of the impact it has on people's well-being, and action taken to address it.

## Chapter summary

- In this chapter, we have looked at some of the terminology associated with mental distress, racism, and cultural diversity, and explored its context.
- We have considered the factors, including the COVID-19 pandemic, that impact on the well-being of people with MH issues who are from minority backgrounds.
- Activities have shown how theories can be used to inform ethical practice, and we have explored how you can ensure best practice when working with people from minority communities with MH issues.

# Activities: brief outline answers

## Activity 8.2   Critical reflection (p160)

First, it is more respectful of others' clinical opinion not to rush to judgement as they might be absolutely correct but just expressing themselves poorly. However, you could probe and ask why they think that, and note that talking therapy would normally be recommended here. A short conversation should let you know where things stand.

If you think that a service user is being denied services based on racism or discrimination, you need to report it. It may be that you have the kind of relationship with your colleague where you can talk to them about things privately and raise your concern. If that is not the case, you will need to speak to your line manager; if you are not satisfied with the response, follow your reporting procedure, and seek support from your union if need be.

The best solution would be a strong service user advocacy presence in your service from the start and clear pathways that are transparent and available to all, so that service users are aware of their options and can more fully participate in their care. When we write our notes, hand them over to colleagues or express professional opinions, we need to be clear that our goal is only to support that individual in recovery – our prejudices are not helpful in doing that, and our first duty is always to the people we treat.

## Activity 8.3   Reflection (p163)

*What factors contributed to the conversation becoming confused?*

You may have answers that are not listed below; it's not an exhaustive list, but there seem to have been a number of misconceptions and misunderstandings.

The first is around translation; getting people who can translate in practice can be tricky, but there are telephone and online services that can help. There are also gender and age dynamics to consider; at 15 years, Hibaq's grandson is still legally a child. He is also male, and both of these factors may affect what Hibaq is comfortable saying in front of him. You should consider managing any pressure on him in this interaction. It is also a mistake to assume that people speak the same language and specific dialects as their family members.

The second point is about beliefs around illness. Mrs Yasin came to the appointment anxious and fearful; these emotions should be addressed as they can impact on communication. She has described her symptomology using strong imagery and by demonstrating physically – unfortunately, these visuals have provoked surprise rather than understanding! There are expectations of formal interactions that differ between people; we only usually consider them when one party steps outside them. Mrs Yasin has been well for many years, and while there is no reason to assume postnatal depression would be followed up 40 years later by psychosis, it is interesting that a past history of mental distress can colour any new assessment. It is also notable that Mrs Yasin did not see her postnatal depression as a mental health issue, but as a social one to do with being newly arrived in a new situation and isolated from former systems of support. As she received her care while in maternity services, it is likely that she thinks she hasn't had contact with MH workers.

> *What could you do to give good care in a situation such as this?*

Ensure that you follow best practice guidance when using an interpreter and be mindful of the things that can go wrong.

Be respectful and friendly – therapeutic communication can be complicated and run into problems but developing warmth and trust in your interactions will only help.

Be aware of body language and verbal cues – if you sense that someone doesn't understand you, stop and clarify. People may use different ways of displaying fear, sadness, and anger, and in some cases physical expression of this kind is frowned upon, so always check!

## Further reading

**Haith, M** (2018) *Understanding Mental Health Practice.* London: Learning Matters.

This book outlines the fundamentals of mental healthcare, equipping you with essential knowledge of what is meant by mental health and well-being, common mental health problems, and typical interventions and treatment options.

**Trenoweth, S** (2022) *Understanding Mental Health Practice for Adult Nursing Students.* London: Learning Matters.

This book gives practical guidance to non-MH trained healthcare professionals on how to respond to the needs of those in your care who face MH challenges, helping you be more prepared and able to deliver person-centred care confidently.

**Younis, T** (2021) The muddle of institutional racism in mental health [Commentary]. *Sociology of Health and Illness*, 43(8): 1831–39.

This journal article takes a thorough look at the complexities of racism, politics, policy, and MH.

## Useful websites

Race Equality Foundation:

**https://raceequalityfoundation.org.uk**

Mental Health UK. Black, Asian, and Minority Ethnic mental health:

**https://mentalhealth-uk.org/black-asian-and-minority-ethnic-bame-mental-health/**

Mind. Existing inequalities have made the mental health of BAME groups worse during the pandemic:

**www.mind.org.uk/news-campaigns/news/existing-inequalities-have-made-mental-health-of-bame-groups-worse-during-pandemic-says-mind/**

Mental Health Foundation. Black, Asian, and Minority Ethnic (BAME) communities:

**www.mentalhealth.org.uk/explore-mental-health/a-z-topics/black-asian-and-minority-ethnic-bame-communities**

# References

Acheson, D (1988) *Public Health in England: The Report of the Committee of Inquiry into the Future Development of the Public Health Function.* London: HMSO.

Al Shamsi, H, Almutairi, AG, Al Mashrafi, S, and Al Kalbani, T (2020) Implications of language barriers for healthcare: a systematic review. *Oman Medical Journal,* 35(2): e122.

Ali, M (2017) Communication skills 1: benefits of effective communication for patients. *Nursing Times,* 113(12): 18–19.

Ali, M (2018) Communication skills 3: non-verbal communication. *Nursing Times,* 114 (2): 41–2.

Almaturi, AF and Rodney, P (2013) Critical cultural competence for culturally diverse workforces. Toward equitable and peaceful healthcare. *Advances in Nursing Science,* 36 (3): 200–12.

Anakwenze, O (2020) The aversive impact of stigma on black people diagnosed with schizophrenia (Doctoral dissertation, Fordham University).

Andrews, N, Greenfield, S, Drever, W, and Redwood, S (2017) Strong, female and black: stereotypes of African Caribbean women's body shape and their effects on clinical encounters. *Health,* 21(2): 189–204.

Argyle, M, Salter, V, Nicholson, H, Williams, M, and Burgess, P (1970) The communication of inferior and superior attitudes by verbal and non-verbal signals. *British Journal of Social and Clinical Psychology,* 9: 221–31.

Assessment, JSN (2022) Public health evidence reports. Available at: https://www. birmingham.gov.uk/downloads/file/24513/trans_community_profile_external_ engagement_presentation (accessed 18 February 2023).

Babbar, P, Shah, P, Abelson, B, and Rhee, AC (2020) Disorders of sexual development in CA Ferrando, *Comprehensive Care of the Transgender Patient* (pp. 25 –33).Elsevier: Amsterdam

Bach, S and Grant, A (2015) *Communication and Interpersonal Skills in Nursing* (3rd edn). London: SAGE.

Bachmann, CL and Gooch, R (2019) *LGBT in Britain: Health Report.* Available at: www. stonewall.org.uk/lgbt-britain-health (accessed 6 October 2019).

Bagci, H and Cinar Yucel, S (2020). A Systematic Review of the Studies about Therapeutic Touch after the Year 2000. *International Journal of Caring Sciences,* 13(1).

Baggott, R (2011) *Public Health Policy and Politics.* London: Palgrave Macmillan.

Baird, J, Yogeswaran, G, Oni, G, and Wilson, EE (2021) What can be done to encourage women from Black, Asian and Minority Ethnic backgrounds to attend breast screening? A qualitative synthesis of barriers and facilitators. *Public Health*, 190: 152–9.

Baker, M (2016) Detecting pressure damage in people with darkly pigmented skin. *Wound Essentials*, 11(1): 28–31.

Bamford, J, Klabbers, G, Curran, E, Rosato, M, and Leavey, G (2021). Social capital and mental health among Black and Minority Ethnic groups in the UK. *Journal Of Immigrant and Minority Health*, 23(3): 502–10.

Barrett, D, Wilson, B, and Woollands, A (2019) *Care Planning: A Guide for Nurses* (3rd edn). London: Routledge.

Baxter, C (1988) *The Black Nurse: An Endangered Species*. Cambridge: National Extension College for Training in Health and Race.

BBC News (2018) *Restrictions Lifted on Dartford Nurse Who Gave Bible to Patient*. Available at: www.bbc.co.uk/news/uk-england-kent-45115124 (accessed 1 June 2019).

Benbow, SM and Kingston, P (2022). Older trans individuals' experiences of health and social care and the views of healthcare and social care practitioners: 'they hadn't a clue'. *Educational Gerontology*, 1–14.

Bentley, GR (2020). Don't blame the BAME: Ethnic and structural inequalities in susceptibilities to COVID-19. *American Journal of Human Biology*, 32(5): e23478. p1–5.

Birthrights (2022) Protecting human rights in childbirth. Systemic racism, not broken bodies. An inquiry into racial injustice and human rights in UK maternity care. Executive summary. Available at: Birthrights-inquiry-systemic-racism_exec-summary_May-22-web. pdf (accessed 6 June 2022).

Bjarnason, D, Mick, J, Thompson, JA, and Cloyd, E (2009) Perspectives on transcultural care. *Nursing Clinics*, 44(4): 495–503.

Bloomfield, J and Pegram, A (2015) Care, compassion and communication. *Nursing Standard*, 29(25): 45–50.

Bonakdar Tehrani, M, Kemp, L, and Baird, K (2022). Culturally and linguistically diverse mothers accessing public health nursing: A narrative review. *Public Health Nursing*, 39(1): 82–8.

Booker, CL, Rieger, G, and Unger, JB (2017) Sexual orientation health inequality: evidence from *Understanding Society*, the UK longitudinal household study. *Preventive Medicine*, 101: 126–32.

Bowers, L, James, K, Quirk, A, Simpson, A, Stewart, D, and Hodsoll, J (2015) Reducing conflict and containment rates on acute psychiatric wards: the Safewards cluster randomised controlled trial. *International Journal of Nursing Studies*, 52(9): 1412–22.

Bränström, R and Pachankis, JE (2020) Reduction in mental health treatment utilization among transgender individuals after gender-affirming surgeries: a total population study. *American Journal of Psychiatry*, 177(8): 727–34.

Bristowe, K, Hodson, M, Wee, B, Almack, K, Johnson, K, Daveson, BA, et al. (2018) Recommendations to reduce inequalities for LGBT people facing advanced illness: ACCESSCare national qualitative interview study. *Palliative Medicine*, 32(1): 23–35.

British Broadcasting Corporation (BBC) (2021) Evan Smith inquest: Hospital 'failure' led to sepsis patient's death. Available at: www.bbc.co.uk/news/uk-england-london-56647361 (accessed 31 January 2022).

Brown, Y (2022) Starting over: Reflections of black men who leave mental health institutions to return to the community. Available at: www.researchgate.net/publication/364785275_Starting_Over_Reflections_of_Black_Men_who_leave_Mental_Health_Institutions_and_Return_to_the_Community (accessed 16 February 2023).

Bucknor-Ferron, P and Zagaja, L (2016) Five strategies to combat unconscious bias. *Nursing*, 46(11): 61–2.

Bunbury, S (2019) Unconscious bias and the medical model: How the social model may hold the key to transformative thinking about disability discrimination. *International Journal of Discrimination and the Law*, 19(1): 26–47.

Burchardt, T, Obolenskaya, P, Vizard, P, and Battaglini, M (2018) *Experience of Multiple Disadvantage among Roma, Gypsy and Traveller Children in England and Wales*. London: LSE.

Burford, B, Worrow, E, and Caspary, A (2009) *Religion or Belief: A Practical Guide for the NHS*. London: Department of Health.

Burnard, P and Gill, P (2014) *Culture, Communication and Nursing*. London: Routledge.

Burnham, J, Palmer, DA, and Whitehouse, L (2008) Learning as a context for differences and differences as a context for learning. *Journal of Family Therapy and Systemic Practice*, 30: 529–42.

Burrell, RR (2019) The black majority church: Exploring the impact of faith and a faith community on mental health and well-being (Doctoral dissertation, Middlesex University/Metanoia Institute).

Burrell, A, and Selman, LE (2022) How do funeral practices impact bereaved relatives' mental health, grief and bereavement? A mixed methods review with implications for COVID-19. *OMEGA – Journal of Death and Dying*, 85(2): 345–83. Available at: https://doi.org/10.1177/0030222820941296 (accessed 16 February 2023).

Buser, JM, Bakari, A, Seidu, AA, Osei-Akoto, A, Paintsil, V, Amoah, R, … and Moyer, CA (2021) Caregiver perception of sickle cell disease stigma in Ghana: an ecological approach. *Journal of Pediatric Health Care*, 35(1): 84–90.

Butler, R (2022) *Vaccine Hesitancy: What It Means and What We Need to Know in Order to Tackle It*. Available at: www.who.int/immunization/research/forums_and_initiatives/1_RButler_VH_Threat_Child_Health_gvirf16.pdf?ua=1 (accessed 6 June 2022).

Byrne, A, Barber, R, and Lim, CH (2021) Impact of the COVID-19 pandemic–a mental health service perspective. *Progress in Neurology and Psychiatry*, 25(2): 27–33b.

Cai, DY (2016) A concept analysis of cultural competence. *International Journal of Nursing Sciences*, 3(3): 268–73.

Cairns, C (2021) *HIV Testing and Prevention Services Affected Badly by COVID in Europe, HIV Treatment Less So*. Available at: www.aidsmap.com/news/nov-2021/hiv-testing-and-prevention-services-affected-badly-covid-europe-hiv-treatment-less-so (accessed 11 February 2023).

Campinha-Bacote, J (2002) The process of cultural competence in the delivery of healthcare services: a model of care. *Journal of Transcultural Nursing*, 13(3): 181–4.

Canada Public Health Association (2016) Public Health Leadership for Action on Health Equity: A Literature Review. Available at: https://nccdh.ca/images/uploads/comments/Public_health_leadership_for_action_on_health_equity_-_A_literature_review_EN_Final.pdf (accessed 18 February 2023).

Cancer Research UK (2020) Breast cancer in men. Available at: www.cancerresearchuk.org/about-cancer/breast-cancer/stages-types-grades/types/male-breast-cancer (accessed 6 June 2022).

Caraher, M, Lloyd, S, and Madelin, T (2014) The 'school foodshed': schools and fast-food outlets in a London borough. *British Food Journal*, 116(3): 472–93.

Caraher, M and Perry, I (2017) Sugar, salt, and the limits of self-regulation in the food industry. *BMJ*, 357: j1709.

Centre for Ageing Better (2022) Summary. The State of Ageing 2022 Report. Available at: https://ageing-better.org.uk/sites/default/files/2022-04/The-State-of-Ageing-2022-online.pdf (accessed 28 May 2022).

Chadwick, L (2022) Mandatory vaccines: Which countries in Europe are making people get the COVID jab? *Euronews*. Available at: www.euronews.com/my-europe/2022/02/01/are-countries-in-europe-are-moving-towards-mandatory-vaccination (accessed 16 February 2023).

Chaffee, MW, Mason, DJ, and Leavitt, JK (2012) A framework for action in policy and politics. In DJ Mason, JK Leavitt, and MW Chaffee (eds), *Policy and Politics in Nursing and Healthcare* (6th edn). St Louis, MO: Elsevier Saunders.

Clark, F (2014) Discrimination against LGBT people triggers health concerns. *The Lancet*, 383(9916): 500–2.

Clarke, J (2016) Spiritual care. In D Sellman and P Snelling (eds), *Becoming a Nurse: Fundamentals of Professional Practice for Nursing*. London: Routledge.

Clarridge, A (2017) Spirituality: a neglected aspect of care. In S Chilton, H Bain, A Clarridge and K Melling (eds), *A Textbook of Community Nursing* (2nd edn). London: Routledge.

Cluley, V (2018) From 'Learning disability to intellectual disability'—Perceptions of the increasing use of the term 'intellectual disability' in learning disability policy, research and practice. *British Journal of Learning Disabilities*, 46: 24–32.

Codjoe, L, Barber, S, and Thornicroft, G (2019) Tackling inequalities: a partnership between mental health services and black faith communities. *Journal of Mental Health*, 28(3): 225–8.

Collins, PH and Bilge, S (2016) *Intersectionality*. Hoboken, NJ: John Wiley & Sons.

Commission on Race and Ethnic Disparities (CRED) (2021) *The Report of the Commission on Race and Ethnic Disparities*. Available at: www.gov.uk/government/publications/the-report-of-the-commission-on-race-and-ethnic-disparities (accessed 10 November 2022).

Cooper, J, Steeg, S, Webb, R, Stewart, SL, Applegate, E, Hawton, K et al. (2013) Risk factors associated with repetition of self-harm in Black and Minority Ethnic (BME) groups: a multi-centre cohort study. *Journal of Affective Disorders*, 148(2): 435–39.

Corless, L, Buckley, A, and Mee, S (2016) Patient narratives 3: Power inequality between patients and nurses. *Nursing Times*, 112(12–13): 20–1.

Coupland, T (2023) Parity of esteem. in C Gamble and G Brennan (eds) *Working with Serious Mental Illness: A Manual for Clinical Practice* (p.107). Oxford: Elsevier.

Corner, L (2019) Reclaiming the word 'queer': what does it mean in 2019? *Gay Times*. Available at https://www.gaytimes.co.uk/life/reclaiming-the-word-queer-what-does-it-mean-in-2019/ (accessed 11 February 2023).

Crenshaw, K (1989) Demarginalizing the intersection of race and sex: A black feminist critique of antidiscrimination doctrine, feminist theory and antiracist politics. *University of Chicago Legal Forum*, 1(8): 139–67.

Cromarty, H (2018) *Gypsies and Travellers*. Briefing Paper, House of Commons Library, Number 08083, 8 May 2018. Available at: https://researchbriefings.parliament.uk/ResearchBriefing/Summary/CBP-8083 (accessed 29 September 2019).

Culley, L (2010) Exclusion and inclusion: unequal lives and unequal health. *Journal of Research in Nursing*, 15(4): 299–301.

Dahl, A and Killen, M (2018). Moral reasoning: Theory and research in developmental science. In J Wixted and S Ghetti (eds), *Stevens' Handbook of Experimental Psychology and Cognitive Neuroscience. Vol. 4: Developmental and Social Psychology* (4th edn, pp. 323–56). New York: Wiley.

Danso, A and Danso, Y (2021) The complexities of race and health. *Future Healthcare Journal*, 8(1): 22.

Department of Health (2005) *Delivering Race Equality in Mental Health Care: An Action Plan For Reform Inside and Outside Services and the Government's Response to the Independent Inquiry into the Death of David Bennett*. Available at: http://webarchive.nationalarchives.gov.uk/20130107105354/http:/www.dh.gov.uk/en/publicationsandstatistics/publications/publicationspolicyandguidance/dh_4100773 (accessed 2 May 2017).

Department of Health (2011) *No Health without Mental Health: A Cross-Government Mental Health Outcomes Strategy for People of All Ages*. Available at: www.gov.uk/government/uploads/system/uploads/attachment_data/file/213761/dh_124058.pdf (accessed 2 May 2017).

Department of Health (2012) *Transforming Care: A National Response to Winterbourne View Hospital: Department of Health Review Final Report*. Available at: https://assets.publishing.service.gov.uk/government/uploads/system/uploads/attachment_data/file/213215/final-report.pdf (accessed 8 January 2022).

Department of Health (2013) *Report of the Mid Staffordshire NHS Foundation Trust Public Enquiry Volume 3: Present and Future*. Available at: https://assets.publishing.service.gov.uk/government/uploads/system/uploads/attachment_data/file/279121/0898_iii.pdf (accessed 13 September 2018).

DeWilde, C and Burton, W (2017) Cultural distress: An emerging paradigm. *Journal of Transcultural Nursing*, 28(4): 334–41.

DHSC (2020) Tackling obesity: empowering adults and children to live healthier lives. Available at: www.gov.uk (accessed 4 November 2022).

DHSC (2021) *Restricting Promotions of Products High in Fat, Sugar and Salt: Consultation Response on Policy Enforcement.* Available at: www.gov.uk/government/consultations/restricting-promotions-of-products-high-in-fat-sugar-and-salt-enforcement/outcome/restricting-promotions-of-products-high-in-fat-sugar-and-salt-consultation-response-on-policy-enforcement (accessed 10 February 2021).

Diabetes UK (2017) How to make reasonable adjustments to diabetes care for adults with a learning disability. *Diabetes UK, London.* Available at: www.diabetes.org.uk/resources-s3/2018-02/Diabetes%20UK%20-%20How%20to%20make%20reasonable%20adjustments%20to%20diabetes%20care%20for%20adults%20with%20a%20learning%20disability.pdf (accessed 10 November 2022).

Diabetes UK (2021) Diabetes diagnoses double in the last 15 years. Available at: www.diabetes.org.uk/about_us/news/diabetes-diagnoses-doubled-prevalence-2021 (accessed 10 February 2021).

Diaz, A, Baweja, R, Bonatakis, JK, and Baweja, R (2021) Global health disparities in vulnerable populations of psychiatric patients during the COVID-19 pandemic. *World Journal of Psychiatry*, 11(4): 94.

Dodd, E, Pracownik, R, Popel, S, Collings, S, Emmens, T, and Cheston, R (2022) Dementia services for people from Black, Asian and Minority Ethnic and White-British communities: Does a primary care based model contribute to equality in service provision? *Health & Social Care in the Community*, 30(2): 622–30.

Dovidio, JF, Esses, VM, Glick, P, and Hewstone, M (2010) *The SAGE Handbook of Prejudice, Stereotyping and Discrimination.* London: SAGE.

Drewniak, D, Krones, T, and Wild, V (2017) Do attitudes and behaviour of health care professionals exacerbate health care disparities among immigrant and ethnic minority groups? An integrative literature review. *International Journal of Nursing Studies*, 70: 89–98.

Dyer, C (2018) *NHS Failed to Communicate Feeding Advice to Refugee Mother, Court Rules.* Available at: www.bmj.com/content/361/bmj.k1711 (accessed 28 April 2018).

Ee, J, Stenfert Kroese, B, and Rose, J (2021). A systematic review of the knowledge, attitudes and perceptions of health and social care professionals towards people with learning disabilities and mental health problems. *British Journal of Learning Disabilities.* Available at: https://doi.org/10.1111/bld.12401

Emerson, E, Hatton, C, Baines, S, and Robertson, J (2016) The physical health of British adults with intellectual disability: cross sectional study. *International Journal for Equity in Health*, 15(1): 11.

Equality Act (2010) *Equality Act 2010: Guidance.* Available at: www.gov.uk/guidance/equality-act-2010-guidance (accessed 5 September 2019).

Equality and Human Rights Commission (EHRC) (2016a) *England's Most Disadvantaged Groups: Gypsies, Travellers and Roma.* Available at: www.equalityhumanrights.com/sites/default/files/is-england-fairer-2016-most-disadvantaged-groups-gypsies-travellers-roma.pdf (accessed 25 October 2019).

Equality and Human Rights Commission (EHRC) (2016b) *Healing a Divided Britain: The Need for a Comprehensive Race Strategy.* Available at: www.equalityhumanrights.com/en/publication-download/healing-divided-britain-need-comprehensive-race-equality-strategy (accessed 9 December 2019).

Equality and Human Rights Commission (EHRC) (2017) *Gypsies and Travellers: Simple Solutions for Living Together.* Available at: www.equalityhumanrights.com/en/gypsies-and-travellers-simple-solutions-living-together (accessed 14 August 2018).

ESRC (2021) Nudging behaviour. Available at: https://esrc.ukri.org/about-us/50-years-of-esrc/50-achievements/nudging-behaviour/ (accessed 10 February 2021).

Essex, R, Markowski, M, and Miller, D (2022) Structural injustice and dismantling racism in health and healthcare. *Nursing Inquiry*, 29(1): e12441–n/a. Available at: https://doi.org/10.1111/nin.12441

Everett, JS, Budescu, M, and Sommers, MS (2012) Making sense of skin color in clinical care. *Clinical Nursing Research*, 21(4): 495–516.

Fafunwa, AB (2018). *History of Education in Nigeria.* London: Routledge.

Farber, JE (2019) Cultural competence of baccalaureate nurse faculty: Relationship to cultural experiences. *Journal of Professional Nursing*, 35: 81–8.

Fardin, MA (2020) COVID-19 and Anxiety: A Review of Psychological Impacts of Infectious Disease Outbreaks. *Arch Clin Infect Dis*, 15 (COVID-19): e102779.

Fenton, K (2016) *Working Globally to Tackle Non-Communicable Diseases.* Available at: https://publichealthmatters.blog.gov.uk/2016/02/09/working-globally-to-tackle-non-communicable-diseases/ (accessed 3 April 2019).

Fernando, S (2003) *Cultural Diversity, Mental Health and Psychiatry: The Struggle against Racism.* Hove: Brunner-Routledge.

Fernando, S (2010) *Mental Health: Race and Culture* (3rd edn). London: Palgrave Macmillan.

Fernando, S and Keating, F (eds) (2009) *Mental Health in a Multi-Ethnic Society: A Multidisciplinary Handbook* (2nd edn). London: Routledge.

FitzGerald, C and Hurst, S (2017) Implicit bias in healthcare professionals: a systematic review. *BMC Medical Ethics*, 18(1): 19.

Flowers, D (2014) *Culturally Competent Nursing Care: A Challenge for the 21st Century.* Available at: http://citeseerx.ist.psu.edu/viewdoc/download?doi=10.1.1.571.300&rep=rep1&type=pdf (accessed 2 September 2019).

Foronda, C (2020) A theory of cultural humility. *Journal of Transcultural Nursing* 31(1): 7–12 https://doi.org/10.1177/1043659619875184 (accessed 16 November 2022).

Foronda, C, MacWilliams, B, and McArthur, E (2016) Interprofessional communication in healthcare: An integrative review. *Nurse Educational Practice*, 19: 36–40.

Forrester-Jones, R (2020) Impact of austerity. Available at: www.Sscr.Nihr.Ac.Uk/Impact-Of-Austerity/ (accessed 8 February 2022).

Foundation for People with Learning Disabilities (2019) *Learning Disability Statistics: Mental Health Problems.* Available at: www.mentalhealth.org.uk/learning-disabilities/help-information/learning-disability-statistics-/187699 (accessed 30 June 2019).

Fredrickson, GM (2015) Models of American ethnic relations: a historical perspective. In *Diverse Nations: Explorations in the History of Racial and Ethnic Pluralism.* London: Routledge.

Fronda, C, Baptiste, D, Reinholdt, MM, and Ousman, K (2016) Cultural Humility: A Concept Analysis. *Journal of Transcultural Nursing*, 27(3): 210–17.

Frost, DM (2011) Social stigma and its consequences for the socially stigmatized. *Social and Personality Psychology Compass*, 5(11): 824–39.

Fuchshuber, P and Greif, W (2022) Creating effective communication and teamwork for patient safety. In *The SAGES Manual of Quality, Outcomes and Patient Safety* (pp. 443–60). Cham: Springer.

Fukada, M (2018) Nursing competency: Definition, structure and development. *Yonago Acta Medica*, 61: 1–7.

Gandy, M (2003) Life without germs: contested episodes in the history of tuberculosis. In M Gandy and A Zumla (eds), *The Return of the White Plague.* London: Verso.

Garner, S (2017) *Racism: An Introduction* (2nd edn). London: SAGE.

General Medical Council (GMC) (2022) Treatment and care towards the end of life: good practice in decision-making. Available at: www.gmc-uk.org/-/media/documents/treatment-and-care-towards-the-end-of-life—english-1015_pdf-48902105.pdf (accessed 23 June 2022).

Giddens, A and Sutton, PW (2017) *Sociology* (8th edn). Cambridge: Polity Press.

Giger, J and Davidhizar, R (2002) The Giger and Davidhizar transcultural assessment model. *Journal of Transcultural Nursing*, 13: 185–8.

Gilbert, L, Teravainen, A, Clark, A, and Shaw, S (2018) *Literacy and Life Expectancy: An Evidence Review Exploring the Link between Literacy and Life Expectancy in England through Health and Socioeconomic Factors.* London: National Literacy Trust.

Gill, P, MacLeod, U, Lester, H, and Hegenbarth, A (2013) *Improving Access to Health Care for Gypsies and Travellers, Homeless People and Sex Workers: An Evidence-Based Commissioning Guide for Clinical Commissioning Groups and Health & Wellbeing Boards.* Available at: www.gypsy-traveller.org/wp-content/uploads/2017/03/RCGP-Social-Inclusion-Commissioning-Guide.pdf (accessed 16 August 2018).

Glasper, A (2016) Ensuring optimal health care for LGBT patients. *British Journal of Nursing*, 25(13): 768–9.

Gleeson, J, Hemmingway, A, and Rosser, E (2015) To what extent do health visitors and school nurses have a voice in the policy process? *Community Practitioner*, 88 (June): 38–41.

Golden, SH (2021) The contribution of structural racism to metabolic health disparities in the USA. *The Lancet Diabetes & Endocrinology*, 9, 478–80.

Golden, S, Brown, A, Cauley, J, Chin, M, Gary-Webb, T, Kim, C et al. (2012) Health disparities in endocrine disorders: biological, clinical, and nonclinical factors – an Endocrine Society scientific statement. *The Journal of Clinical Endocrinology and Metabolism*, 97(9): E1579–639.

GOV.UK (2021) *New Every Mind Matters Campaign To Improve People's Mental Health*. Available at: www.gov.uk/government/news/new-every-mind-matters-campaign-to-improve-peoples-mental-health (accessed 10 November 2022).

GOV.UK (2019) *Public Mental Health*. Available at: www.gov.uk/government/collections/public-mental-health#improving-the-lives-of-people-with-mental-health-problems (accessed 1 November 2022).

Government Equalities Office (2018) *National LGBT Survey Summary Report*. Available at: https://assets.publishing.service.gov.uk/government/uploads/system/uploads/attachment_data/file/722314/GEO-LGBT-Survey-Report.pdf (accessed 20 August 2019).

Green, MA, Evans, CR, and Subramanian, SV (2017) Can intersectionality theory enrich population health research? *Social Science & Medicine*, 178: 214–26.

Greenfields, M (2017) Good practice in working with Gypsy, Traveller and Roma communities. *Primary Health Care*, 27(10): 24–9.

Griffith, JK (2009) *The Religious Aspect of Nursing Care*. Available at: https://nursing.ubc.ca/sites/nursing.ubc.ca/files/documents/ReligiousAspectsofNursingCareEEdition.pdf (accessed 2 September 2019).

Guardian Press Association (2011) *Nurse Jailed for Killing Her Baby by Force-Feeding*. Available at: www.theguardian.com/uk/2011/nov/11/nurse-jailed-baby-force-feeding (accessed 1 August 2018).

Gurdasani, D, Barroso, I, Zeggini, E et al. (2019) Genomics of disease risk in globally diverse populations. *Nat Rev Genet*, 20: 520–35. Available at: https://doi.org/10.1038/s41576-019-0144-0 (accessed 16 February 2023).

Gysbertha, F (2023) 'We're seen as human after we're dead': Exploring Black men's barriers to expressing psychological distress. Doctoral dissertation, Norwich: University of East London.

Hamed, S, Thapar-Björkert, S, Bradby, H, and Ahlberg, BM (2020) Racism in European health care: structural violence and beyond. *Qualitative Health Research*, 30(11): 1662–73.

Haney, AM and Rollock, D (2018) A matter of faith: The role of religion, doubt, and personality in emerging adult mental health. *Psychology of Religion and Spirituality*. Advance online publication.

Harvard Health Publishing (2021) *What Is Neurodiversity?* Available at: /www.health.harvard.edu/blog/what-is-neurodiversity-202111232645 (accessed 11 February 2023).

Hastings, A, Bailey, N, Bramley, G, and Gannon, M (2017) Austerity urbanism in England: the 'regressive redistribution' of local government services and the impact on the poor and marginalised. *Environment and Planning A: Economy and Space*, 49(9): 2007–24.

Hatton, C, Emerson, E, Robertson, J, and Baines, S (2017) The mental health of British adults with intellectual impairments living in general households. *Journal of Applied Research in Intellectual Disabilities*, 30(1): 188–97.

Hawthorne, DM and Gordon, SC (2020) The invisibility of spiritual nursing care in clinical practice. *Journal of Holistic Nursing*, 38(1): 147–55.

Hayanga, B, Stafford, M, Saunders, CL, and Bécares, L (2022) Ethnic inequalities in age-related patterns of multiple long-term conditions in England: Analysis of primary care and nationally representative survey data. Available at: https://doi.org/10.1101/2022.03.31.22273224

Haywood, C, Lanzkron, S, Bediako, S, Strouse, JJ, Haythornthwaite, J, Carroll, CP et al. (2014) Perceived discrimination, patient trust, and adherence to medical recommendations among persons with sickle cell disease. *Journal of General Internal Medicine*, 29(12): 1657–62.

Health Education England (2018) *Diversity and Inclusion: Our Strategic Framework 2018–2022*. Available at: www.hee.nhs.uk/sites/default/files/documents/Diversity%20and%20Inclusion%20-%20Our%20Strategic%20Framework.pdf (accessed 6 October 2019).

Health Foundation (2018) *What Makes Us Healthy? An Introduction to Social Determinants of Health*. Available at: www.health.org.uk/sites/default/files/What-makes-us-healthy-quick-guide.pdf (accessed 28 September 2019).

Heaslip, V (2015) Caring for people from diverse cultures. *British Journal of Community Nursing*, 20(9): 421.

Helman, CG (2007) *Culture, Health and Illness* (5th edn). London: Hodder Arnold.

Henderson, S, Horne, M, Hills, R, and Kendall, E (2018) Cultural competence in healthcare in the community: a concept analysis. *Health and Social Care in the Community*, 26(4): 590–603, https://doi.org/10.1111/hsc.12556.

Heslop, P, Blair, PS, Fleming, P, Hoghton, M, Marriott, A, and Russ, L (2014) The Confidential Inquiry into premature deaths of people with intellectual disabilities in the UK: A population-based study. *The Lancet*, 383: 889–95.

HM Government (2013) *Equality Act 2010: Guidance*. Available at: www.gov.uk/guidance/equality-act-2010-guidance (accessed 5 September 2019).

HM Treasury (2015) *Soft Drinks Industry Levy Comes into Effect*. Available at: www.gov.uk/government/news/soft-drinks-industry-levy-comes-into-effect (accessed 4 September 2019).

Holland, L and Ousey, K (2011) Inclusion or exclusion: Recruiting Black and Minority Ethnic community individuals as simulated patients. *Ethnicity and Inequalities in Health and Social Care*, 4(2): 81–90.

Holm, AL, Gorosh, MR, Brady, M, and White-Perkins, D (2017) Recognizing privilege and bias: An interactive exercise to expand health care providers' personal awareness. *Academic Medicine*, 92(3): 360–4.

House of Commons Women and Equalities Committee (2016) Transgender equality: First report of session 2015–2016. London: The Stationery Office (HC390). Available at: www.publications.parliament.uk/pa/cm201516/cmselect/cmwomeq/390/39003.htm#_idTextAnchor216 (accessed 8 August 2022).

House of Commons, and Health and Social Care and Science and Technology Committees (2021) Coronavirus: lessons learned to date. Available at: https://committees.parliament.uk/publications/7496/documents/78687/default/ (accessed 8 January 22).

Hurley, R (2018) Chaplaincy for the 21st century, for people of all religions and none. *British Medical Journal*, 363.

Iacobucci, G (2021) COVID-19 and pregnancy: vaccine hesitancy and how to overcome it. *British Medical Journal*, 375: n2862.

International Diabetes Federation (2020) *Diabetic Retinopathy Barometer Report: Global Findings*. Available at: https://idf.org/our-activities/care-prevention/eye-health/dr-barometer.html (accessed 10 February 2022).

International Lesbian, Gay, Bisexual, Trans and Intersex Association (ILGA) (2020a) *World Trans Legal Mapping Report 2019: Recognition Before the Law*. Geneva: ILGA World.

International Lesbian, Gay, Bisexual, Trans and Intersex Association (ILGA) (2020b) *ILGA World Updates State-Sponsored Homophobia Report: There's Progress in Times of Uncertainty*. Available at: https://ilga.org/ilga-world-releases-state-sponsored-homophobia-December-2020-update (accessed 30 January 2022).

Jandt, FE and Jandt, FE (2018) *An Introduction to Intercultural Communication: Identities in a Global Community* (9th edn). Thousand Oaks: SAGE.

Jannesari, S, Hatch, S, Prina, M, and Oram, S (2020) Post-migration social–environmental factors associated with mental health problems among asylum seekers: A systematic review. *Journal of Immigrant and Minority Health*, 22(5): 1055–64.

Jardine, J, Walker, K, Gurol-Urganci, I, Webster, K, Muller, P, Hawdon, J, Khalil, A, Harris, T, Van Der Meulen, J, and Maternity, N (2021) Adverse pregnancy outcomes attributable to socioeconomic and ethnic inequalities in England: A national cohort study. *The Lancet*, 398: 1905–12.

Jaspal, R and Lopes, B (2021) Discrimination and mental health outcomes in British Black and South Asian people during the COVID-19 outbreak in the UK. *Mental Health, Religion & Culture*, 24(1): 80–96.

Jehovah's Witnesses (2018) *Information on Blood Transfusion Beliefs*. Available at: www.jw.org/en/search/?q=blood+transfusion (accessed 23 August 2018).

Johl, N, Patterson, T, and Pearson, L (2016) What do we know about the attitudes, experiences and needs of Black and Minority Ethnic carers of people with dementia in the United Kingdom? A systematic review of empirical research findings. *Dementia*, 15 (4): 721–42.

Jonassaint, CR, Jones, VL, Leong, S, and Frierson, GM (2016) A systematic review of the association between depression and health care utilization in children and adults with sickle cell disease. *British Journal of Haematology*, 174(1): 136–47.

Jorm, AF, Korten, AE, Jacomb, PA, Christensen, H, Rodgers, B, and Pollitt, P (1997) Mental health literacy: A survey of the public's ability to recognise mental disorders and their belief about the effectiveness of treatment. *Medical Journal of Australia*, 166: 182–6.

Jurcic, M (2016) *Working with Victims of Anti-LGBT Hate Crimes: A Practical Handbook.* Available at: www.galop.org.uk/wp-content/uploads/Working-with-Victims-of-Anti%E2%80%93LGBT-Hate-Crimes.pdf (accessed 7 October 2019).

Kane, E (2014) *Prevalence, Patterns and Possibilities: The Experience of People from Black and Ethnic Minorities with Mental Health Problems in the Criminal Justice System.* Available at: https://3bx16p38bchl32s0e12di03h-wpengine.netdna-ssl.com/wp-content/uploads/2014/05/prevalence-patterns-and-possibilities.pdf (accessed 9 December 2019).

Kapur, N (2015) Unconscious bias harms patients and staff. *BMJ*, 351: h6347.

Katikireddi, SV, Lal, S, Carrol, ED, Niedzwiedz, CL, Khunti, K, Dundas, R, Diderichsen, F, and Barr, B (2021) Unequal impact of the COVID-19 crisis on Minority Ethnic groups: a framework for understanding and addressing inequalities. *J Epidemiol Community Health*, 75(10): 970–4.

Kavanagh, A, Dickinson, H, Carey, G, Llewellyn, G, Emerson, E, Disney, G, and Hatton, C (2021) Improving health care for disabled people in COVID-19 and beyond: lessons from Australia and England. *Disability and Health Journal*, 14(2): 101050.

Kavanagh, A, Hatton, C, Stancliffe, RJ, Aitken, Z, King, T, Hastings, R, … and Emerson, E. (2022) Health and healthcare for people with disabilities in the UK during the COVID-19 pandemic. *Disability and Health Journal*, 15(1): 101171.

Kelsall-Knight, L (2022) Practising cultural humility to promote person and family-centred care. *Nursing Standard*. doi:10.7748/ns.2022.e11880 (accessed 16 November 2022).

Khalaf, IA, Al-Dweik, G, Abu-Snieneh, H, Al-Daken, L, Musallam, RM, BaniYounis, M et al. (2018) Nurses' experiences of grief following patient death: A qualitative approach. *Journal of Holistic Nursing*, 36(3): 228–40.

Killen, M and Dahl, A (2021) Moral Reasoning Enables Developmental and Societal Change. *Perspectives on Psychological Science*, 16(6), 1209–25. Available at: https://doi-org.roe.idm.oclc.org/10.1177/1745691620964076 (accessed 16 November 2022).

Kirkbride, JB, Barker, D, Cowden, F, Stamps, R, Yang, M, Jones, PB et al. (2008) Psychoses, ethnicity and socio-economic status. *British Journal of Psychiatry*, 193(1): 18–24.

Knapp, M (2012) Mental health in an age of austerity. *Evidence-Based Mental Health*, 15(3): 54–5.

Kwame, A and Petrucka, PM (2021) A literature-based study of patient-centered care and communication in nurse-patient interactions: barriers, facilitators, and the way forward. *BMC Nursing*, 20(1): 1–10.

Lagisetty, PA, Priyadarshini, S, Terrell, S, Hamati, M, Landgraf, J, Chopra, V, and Heisler, M (2017) Culturally targeted strategies for diabetes prevention in minority populations: a systematic review and framework. *The Diabetes Educator*, 43(1): 54–77.

Lakkakula, BVKS, Sahoo, R, Verma, H, and Lakkakula, S (2018) Pain management issues as part of the comprehensive care of patients with sickle cell disease. *Pain Manag Nurs*, 19(6): 558–72.

Lalani, N (2020) Meanings and interpretations of spirituality in nursing and health. *Religions*, 11(9): 428.

Lane, P, Spencer, S, McCready, M, and Roddam, M (2019) *Life On and Off of the Hard Shoulder: Older Gypsies living on the Roadside and in Housing*. Cambridge: Anglia Ruskin University, pp. 1–42.

Larsson, P (2013) The rhetoric/reality gap in social determinants of mental health. *Mental Health Review Journal*, 18(4): 182–93.

Lassiter, JM, Saleh, L, Grov, C, Starks, T, Ventuneac, A, and Parsons, JT (2017) Spirituality and multiple dimensions of religion are associated with mental health in gay and bisexual men: results from the One Thousand Strong cohort. *Psychology of Religion and Spirituality*, 11(4): 408–16.

Latif, A, Tariq, S, Abbasi, N, and Mandane, B (2018) Giving voice to the medically under-served: a qualitative co-production approach to explore patient medicine experiences and improve services to marginalized communities. *Pharmacy*, 6(1): 13.

Leininger, M (1978) *Transcultural Nursing: Concepts, Theories and Practices*. New York: John-Wiley.

Leininger, M (1988) Leininger's theory of nursing: Cultural care diversity and universality. *Nursing Science Quarterly*, 1(4): 152–60.

Leininger, M (ed.) (1995) *Transcultural Nursing: Concepts, Theories, Research, And Practices* (2nd edn) (pp. 93–112). New York: McGraw-Hill.

Lekas, H-M, Pahl, K, and Fuller Lewis, C (2020). Rethinking Cultural Competence: Shifting to Cultural Humility. *Health Services Insights*, 13. doi: 10.1177/1178632920970580 (accessed 14 November 2022).

Lexico (2019a) *Communication*. Available at: www.lexico.com/en/definition/coomunication (accessed 21 September 2019).

Lexico (2019b) *Competent*. Available at: www.lexico.com/en/definition/competent (accessed 21 September 2019).

LGBT Foundation (2020) *Hidden Figures: The Impact of the Covid-19 Pandemic on LGBT Communities in the UK* (3rd edn). Available at: https://lgbt.foundation/coronavirus/hiddenfigures

Lim, E, Alexander, N, Hanson, S, Tosich, T, O'Brien, F, Chu, M, and Frotjold, A (2022) Responding to no-visitor policies during the COVID-19 pandemic: Virtual care initiatives for hospitalized patients. *Journal of Advanced Nursing*, 78(4): e62–e63.

Louch, G, Albutt, A, Harlow-Trigg, J et al. (2021) Exploring patient safety outcomes for people with learning disabilities in acute hospital settings: a scoping review. *BMJ Open*, 11: e047102.

Luchenski, S, Magurie, N, Aldridge, R, Hayward, A, Story, A, Perri, P et al. (2018) What works in inclusion health: overview of effective interventions for marginalised and excluded populations. *The Lancet*, 391(10117): 266–80.

Ma, Y, Riaz, A, Shaikh, AM, Bhatti, DS, Farid, M, and Khan, MAA (2022) Exploring the Perceptions Surrounding Hospital Chaplains in Patient Care and Healing. *Journal of Pastoral Care & Counseling*, 76(3): 181–88.

Mabuka-Maroa, J (2019) Africa needs a heavy dose of investment in genomics research. *The Conversation.* Available at: http://theconversation.com/africa-needs-a-heavy-dose-of-investment-in-genomics-research-114456 (accessed 9 December 2019).

MacInnes, P (2020) 'BAME' term offends those it attempts to describe, sporting survey finds. *The Guardian.* Available at: www.theguardian.com/sport/2020/nov/12/bame-term-offends-those-it-attempts-to-describe-sporting-survey-finds-sporting-equals (accessed 16 February 2023).

Mackert, M, Mabry-Flynn, A, Donovan, EE, Champlin, S, and Pounders, K (2019) Health literacy and perceptions of stigma. *Journal of Health Communication*, 24(11): 856–64.

Major, B, Dovidio, JF, and Link, BG (eds) (2017) The Oxford handbook of stigma, discrimination and health. Oxford University Press. Available at: https://doi.org/10.1093/oxfordhb/9780190243470.001.0001 (accessed 7 August 2022).

Malli, AM, Sams, L, Forrester-Jones, R, Murphy, G, and Henwood, M (2018) Austerity and the lives of people with learning disabilities. A thematic synthesis of current literature. *Disability & Society*, 33(9): 1412–35.

Markey, K (2021) Moral reasoning as a catalyst for cultural competence and culturally responsive care. *Nursing Philosophy*, 22: e12337. Available at: https://doi.org/10.1111/nup.12337 (accessed 15 April 2022).

Marks, TV and Vanderslott, S (2021) Which countries have mandatory childhood vaccination policies? Available at: https://ourworldindata.org/childhood-vaccination-policies (accessed 10 January 2022).

Marmot, M (2015) *Fair Society, Healthy Lives: A Strategic Review of Health Inequalities in England Post-2010.* London: UCL.

Marmot, M, Allen J, Boyce, T, Goldblatt, P, and Morrison, J (2020a) *Health Equity in England: The Marmot Review 10 years on, Institute of Health Equity.* Available at: www.health.org.uk/publications/reports/the-marmot-review-10-years-on (accessed 16 February 2023).

Marmot, M, Allen J, Boyce, T, Goldblatt, P, and Morrison, J (2021) *Build Back Fairer in Greater Manchester: Health Equity and Dignified Lives.* Available at: www.instituteofhealthequity.org/resources-reports/build-back-fairer-in-greater-manchester-health-equity-and-dignified-lives/build-back-fairer-in-greater-manchester-executive-summary.pdf (accessed 1 February 2022).

Marmot, M, Allen, J, Goldblatt, P, Boyce, T, McNeish, D, Grady, M et al. (2010) *The Marmot Review: Fair Society, Healthy Lives – The Strategic Review of Health Inequalities in England Post-2010.* London: UCL (accessed 16 February 2023).

Marmot, M, Allen, J, Goldblatt, P, Boyce, T, Mcneish, D, Grady, M, and Geddes, I (2020b) Fair society, healthy lives: the Marmot review. 2010. *Final Report*. Available at: https://doi.org/10.1016/j.puhe.2012.05.014 (accessed 16 February 2023).

Marmot, M, Allen J, Goldblatt, P, and Heard, E (2020c) *Build Back Fairer: The COVID-19 Marmot Review*. Available at www.health.org.uk/publications/build-back-fairer-the-covid-19-marmot-review (accessed 4 June 2022).

MBRRACE-UK (2021) *Saving Lives, Improving Mothers' Care Lessons Learned to Inform Maternity Care from the UK and Ireland Confidential Enquiries into Maternal Deaths and Morbidity 2017–2019*. Available at: www.npeu.ox.ac.uk/assets/downloads/mbrrace-uk/reports/maternal-report-2021/MBRRACE-UK_Maternal_Report_2021_-_FINAL_-_WEB_VERSION.pdf (accessed 31 January 2022).

McCarthy, J, Cassidy, I, Graham, M, and Tuohy, D (2013) Conversations through barriers of language and interpretation. *British Journal of Nursing*, 22(6): 335–9.

McCartney, G, Popham, F, McMaster, R, and Cumbers, A (2019). Defining health and health inequalities. *Public Health*, 172: 1–14.

McConnell, E (2001) Competence vs. competency. *Nursing Management*, 32(5): 14.

McCullough, S (2014) *An Exploration of Political Awareness amongst a Cohort of All Field Students, in One University in Northern Ireland*. Available at: http://pure.qub.ac.uk/portal/files/13229771/Trinity_Dublin_Nov_2014.pptx (accessed 4 September 2019).

McKey, S, Quirke, B, Fitzpatrick, P, Kelleher, C, and Malone, K (2020) A rapid review of Irish Traveller mental health and suicide: A psychosocial and anthropological perspective. *Irish Journal of Psychological Medicine*, 39(2): 223-233. Available at: https://doi.org/10.1017/ipm.2020.108

McManus, S, Meltzer, H, Brugha, T, Bebbington, P, Brugha, T, Coid, J et al. (2009) Adult psychiatric morbidity in England, 2007: results of a household survey. In S McManus, H Meltzer, T Brugha et al. (eds), *The NHS Information Centre for Health and Social Care*. London: NHS.

McSherry, W and Jamieson, S (2011) An online survey of nurses' perceptions of spirituality and spiritual care. *Journal of Clinical Nursing*, 20(11–12): 1757–67.

Meddings, F and Haith-Cooper, M (2008) Culture and communication in ethically appropriate care. *Nursing Ethics*, 15: 52–61.

Memon, A, Taylor, K, Mohebati, LM, Sundin, J, Cooper, M, Scanlon, T et al. (2016) *Perceived Barriers to Accessing Mental Health Services among Black and Minority Ethnic (BME) Communities: A Qualitative Study in Southeast England*. Available at: https://bmjopen.bmj.com/content/bmjopen/6/11/e012337.full.pdf (accessed 1 July 2018).

Mencap (2013) *Mencap Research: 'Scandal of Avoidable Death' as 1,200 People with a Learning Disability Die Needlessly Every Year in NHS Care*. Available at: www.mencap.org.uk/press-release/mencap-research-scandal-avoidable-death-1200-people-learning-disability-die (accessed 6 October 2019).

Mencap (2020) *Mencap Responds to ONS Statistics on the Social Impact of COVID-19 For People with a Disability*. Available at: www.mencap.org.uk/press-release/mencap-responds-ons-statistics-social-impact-covid-19-people-disability (accessed 11 January 2021).

Mencap (2022) *How Common is Learning Disability?* Available at: www.mencap.org.uk/ learning-disability-explained/research-and-statistics/how-common-learning-disability (accessed on 31 January 2022).

Mendes, A (2015) Culture and religion in nursing: providing culturally sensitive care. *British Journal of Nursing*, 24(8): 459.

Mental Health UK (MH, UK) (n.d.) Black, Asian and Minority Ethnic mental health. Available at https://mentalhealth-uk.org/black-asian-and-minority-ethnic-bame-mental-health/

Mereish, EH, Liu, MM and Helms, JE (2012) Effects of discrimination on Chinese, Filipino, and Vietnamese Americans' mental and physical health. *Asian American Journal of Psychology*, 3(2): 91–103.

Mergenthaler, A and Yasseri, T (2021) Selling sex: what determines rates and popularity? An analysis of 11,500 online profiles. *Culture, Health & Sexuality*, 24(7): 935–52.

Milner, A and Jumbe, S (2020) Using the right words to address racial disparities in COVID-19. *Lancet Public Health*, 5(8): e419–20. doi: 10.1016/S2468-2667(20)30162-6. Epub 2020 July 21 Available at: https://pubmed.ncbi.nlm.nih.gov/32707127 (accessed 9 November 2022).

Moore, HE, Siriwardena, AN, Gussy, M, Tanser, F, Hill, B, and Spaight, R (2021). Mental health emergencies and COVID-19: the impact of 'lockdown' in the East Midlands of the UK. *BJPsych Open*, 7(4) e139.

Morgan, C, Abdul-Al, R, Lappin, JM, Jones, P, Fearon, P, Leese, M et al. (2006) Clinical and social determinants of duration of untreated psychosis in the AESOP first-episode psychosis study. *British Journal of Psychiatry*, 189(5): 446–52.

Moro, TT, Savage, TA, and Gehlert, S (2017) Agency, social and healthcare supports for adults with intellectual disability at the end of life in out-of-home, non-institutional community residences in Western nations: a literature review. *Journal of Applied Research in Intellectual Disabilities*, 30(6): 1045–56.

Murji, K and Solomos, J (2015) Conclusion: back to the future. In K Murji and J Solomos (eds), *Theories of Race and Ethnicity: Contemporary Debates and Perspectives*. Cambridge: Cambridge University Press.

Myers, J (2015) Challenges of identifying eczema in darkly pigmented skin. *Nursing Children and Young People*, 27(6): 24–8.

Naidoo, J and Wills, J (eds) (2022) *Health Studies: An Introduction*. Springer Nature.

*Narrative Inquiry in Bioethics Editors* (2014) Introduction: religion in medical and nursing practice. *Narrative Inquiry in Bioethics*, 4(3): 189–90.

National AIDS Trust (2021) *HIV in the UK Statistics*. Available at: www.nat.org.uk/about-hiv/hiv-statistics (accessed 10 January 22).

National Health Service Act (1946) Available at: www.legislation.gov.uk/ukpga/1946/81/ pdfs/ukpga_19460081_en.pdf (accessed 6 October 2019).

National Health Service Race and Health Observatory (2022) *Ethnic Inequalities in Healthcare: A Rapid Evidence Review*. Available at: RHO-Rapid-Review-Final-Report_v.7.pdf (nhsrho.org) (accessed 14 November 2022).

National Literacy Trust (2017) *Adult Literacy*. Available at: https://literacytrust.org.uk/parents-and-families/adult-literacy/ (accessed 7 April 2018).

Nazroo, JY, Bhui, KS, and Rhodes, J (2020) Where next for understanding race/ethnic inequalities in severe mental illness? Structural, interpersonal and institutional racism. *Sociology of Health & Illness*, 42(2), 262–76.

Neale, N and Sale, J (eds) (2022) *Developing Practical Nursing Skills: Foundations for Nursing and Healthcare Students*. London: Routledge.

Nelson, TD (2015) *Handbook of Prejudice, Stereotyping, and Discrimination* (2nd edn). London: Routledge.

*New Scientist* (2021) COVID-19: The story of a pandemic. *New Scientist*, 10 March.

Neve, KL and Isaacs, A (2021) How does the food environment influence people engaged in weight management? A systematic review and thematic synthesis of the qualitative literature. *Obesity Reviews*, e13398.

NHS (2019) *Breast Cancer Screening*. Available at: www.nhs.uk/conditions/breast-cancer-screening/ (accessed 29 August 2019).

NHS Digital (2021) *Health literacy*. Available at https://service-manual.nhs.uk/content/health-literacy (accessed 2 October 2022).

NHS Education for Scotland (2021) *Spiritual Care Matters: An Introductory Resource for all NHS Scotland Staff*. Available at www.nes.scot.nhs.uk/media/xzadagnc/spiritual-care-matters-an-introductory-resource-for-all-nhsscotland-staff.pdf (accessed 21 June 2022).

NHS England (2015) *Introducing the 6Cs*. Available at: www.england.nhs.uk/6cs/wp-content/uploads/sites/25/2015/03/introducing-the-6cs.pdf (accessed 13 November 2019).

NHS England and NHS Improvement (2019) *Reducing Deaths Of People With A Learning Disability in NHS Acute (Hospital) Trusts in England: An Improvement Tool. User Manual*. Available at: www.england.nhs.uk/wpcontent/uploads/2020/08/Reducing_deaths_of_people_with_a_learning_disability__user_manual_.pdf (accessed 31 January 2022).

NHS Health and Social Care Information Centre (2005) *Health Survey for England 2004: The Health of Minority Ethnic Groups*. Available at: https://files.digital.nhs.uk/publicationimport/pub01xxx/pub01209/heal-surv-hea-eth-min-hea-tab-eng-2004-rep.pdf (accessed 3 September 2019).

NHS Improvement (2018) *The Learning Disability Improvement Standards for NHS Trusts*. Available at: https://improvement.nhs.uk/resources/learning-disability-improvement-standards-nhs-trusts/ (accessed 2 December 2018).

NHS Scotland (2019) *Scottish Palliative Care Guidelines: Patient and Family Focus*. Available at: www.palliativecareguidelines.scot.nhs.uk/guidelines/about-the-guidelines/patient-and-family-focus.aspx (accessed 13 October 2019).

NHS Scotland Chaplaincy Services (2007) *Standards for NHS Scotland Chaplaincy Services*. Available at: www.nes.scot.nhs.uk/media/290156/chaplaincy__standards_final_version.pdf (accessed 13 October 2019).

NICE (2016) *HIV Testing: Increasing Uptake Among People Who May Have Undiagnosed HIV.* Available at: www.nice.org.uk/guidance/ng60 (accessed 8 February 2022).

Nolan, TS, Alston, A, Choto, R, and Moss, KO (2021) Cultural Humility: Retraining and retooling nurses to provide equitable cancer care. *Clinical Journal of Oncology Nursing*, 25(5), pp. 3–9. doi: 10.1188/21.CJON.S1.3-9 (accessed 14 November 2022).

Nordenfelt, L (2007) The concepts of health and illness revisited. *Medicine, Health Care and Philosophy*, 10(1): 5–10.

Norouzinia, R, Aghabarari, M, Shiri, M, Karimi, M, and Samami, E (2016) Communication barriers perceived by nurses and patients. *Global Journal of Health Science*, 8(6): 65–74.

NSC NHS Strategic Health Authority (2003) *Independent Inquiry into the Death of David Bennett: An Independent Inquiry Set Up under HSG (94)27.* Available at: www.rbmind.org/DocumentLibrary/DavidBennettEquiry.pdf (accessed 2 May 2017).

Nuffield Council on Bioethics (2007) *Public Health: Ethical Issues.* Available at: www.nuffieldbioethics.org/publications/public-health (accessed 10 January 2022).

Nursing and Midwifery Council (NMC) (2004) *Standards of Proficiency for Specialist Community Public Health Nurses.* Available at: www.nmc.org.uk/globalassets/sitedocuments/standards/nmc-standards-of-proficiency-for-specialist-community-public-health-nurses.pdf (accessed 3 September 2019).

Nursing and Midwifery Council (NMC) (2012) *Conduct and Competence Committee: Substantive Hearing Case Gloria Dwomoh.* Available at: www.nmc.org.uk/globalassets/sitedocuments/ftpoutcomes/2012/october/reasons-dwomoh-cccsh-29808-20121022.pdf (accessed 10 August 2018).

Nursing and Midwifery Council (NMC) (2017) *Enabling Professionalism.* Available at: www.nmc.org.uk/globalassets/sitedocuments/other-publications/enabling-professionalism.pdf (accessed 22 August 2018).

Nursing and Midwifery Council (NMC) (2018a) *Future Nurse: Standards of Proficiency for Registered Nurses.* Available at: www.nmc.org.uk/globalassets/sitedocuments/education-standards/future-nurse-proficiencies.pdf (accessed 25 June 2018).

Nursing and Midwifery Council (NMC) (2018b) *The Code: Professional Standards of Practice and Behaviour for Nurses, Midwives and Nursing Associates.* Available at: www.nmc.org.uk/globalassets/sitedocuments/nmc-publications/nmc-code.pdf.

Nursing and Midwifery Council (NMC) (2018c) *Standards of Proficiency for Registered Nurses.* Available at: Standards of proficiency for registered nurses – The Nursing and Midwifery Council (nmc.org.uk) (accessed 14 November 2022).

Nursing and Midwifery Council (NMC) (2019) *Concerns, Complaints and Referrals.* Available at: www.nmc.org.uk/concerns-nurses-midwives/concerns-complaints-and-referrals/ (accessed 24 October 2019).

Nutbeam, D (2004) Getting evidence into policy and practice to address health inequalities. *Health Promotion International*, 19(2): 137–40.

Nutbeam, D and Muscat, DM (2020). Advancing health literacy interventions. In *Health Literacy in Clinical Practice and Public Health* (pp. 115–27). Amsterdam: IOS Press.

Nyatanga, B (2018) Cultural competence in palliative care and a world of multiculturalism. *British Journal of Community Nursing*, 23(6): 307.

O'Brien, G and Pearson, J (2004) Autism and learning disability. *Autism*, 8(2): 125–40.

O'Hagan, K (2001) *Cultural Competence in the Caring Professions*. London: Jessica Kingsley.

Office for Health Improvement and Disparities (2021) Public health profiles. Available at: https://fingertips.phe.org.uk/profile/public-health-outcomes-framework (accessed 16 February 2023).

Office for National Statistics (ONS) (2017a) *Causes of Death Over 100 Years*. Available at: www.ons.gov.uk/peoplepopulationandcommunity/birthsdeathsandmarriages/deaths/articles/causesofdeathover100years/2017-09-18 (accessed 11 January 2022).

Office for National Statistics (ONS) (2017b) *National Life Tables, UK: 2014 to 2016*. Available at: www.ons.gov.uk/peoplepopulationandcommunity/birthsdeathsandmarriages/lifeexpectancies/bulletins/nationallifetablesunitedkingdom/2014to2016 (accessed 29 August 2019).

Office for National Statistics (ONS) (2018) *Overview of the UK Population: November 2018*. Available at: www.ons.gov.uk/peoplepopulationandcommunity/populationandmigration/populationestimates/articles/overviewoftheukpopulation/november2018 (accessed 3 September 2019).

Office for National Statistics (ONS) (2019a) *Overview of the UK Population: August 2019*. Available at: www.ons.gov.uk/peoplepopulationandcommunity/populationandmigration/populationestimates/articles/overviewoftheukpopulation/august2019/previous/v1 (accessed 29 September 2019).

Office for National Statistics (ONS) (2019b) *Population Estimates for the UK, England and Wales, Scotland and Northern Ireland: Mid-2018*. Available at: www.ons.gov.uk/peoplepopulationandcommunity/populationandmigration/populationestimates/bulletins/annualmidyearpopulationestimates/mid2018 (accessed 5 October 2019).

Office for National Statistics (ONS) (2019c) *Sexual Orientation, UK: 2017*. Available at: www.ons.gov.uk/peoplepopulationandcommunity/culturalidentity/sexuality/bulletins/sexualidentityuk/2017 (accessed 5 October 2019).

Office for National Statistics (ONS) (2019d) *Population Estimates by Ethnic Group and Religion, England and Wales: 2019*. Available at: www.ons.gov.uk/peoplepopulationandcommunity/populationandmigration/populationestimates/articles/populationestimatesbyethnicgroupandreligionenglandandwales/2019

Office for National Statistics (ONS) (2021a) *Population estimates for the UK, England and Wales, Scotland, and Northern Ireland: mid-2020*. Available at: www.ons.gov.uk/peoplepopulationandcommunity/populationandmigration/populationestimates/bulletins/annualmidyearpopulationestimates/latest (accessed 31 January 2022).

Office for National Statistics (ONS) (2021b) *Coronavirus and Vaccine Hesitancy, Great Britain: 9 August 2021*. Available at: www.ons.gov.uk/peoplepopulationandcommunity/healthandsocialcare/healthandwellbeing/bulletins/coronavirusandvaccinehesitancygreatbritain/9august2021 (accessed 10 January 2022).

Office for National Statistics (ONS) (2021c) *Sexual Orientation, UK: 2019.* Available at: www.ons.gov.uk/peoplepopulationandcommunity/culturalidentity/sexuality/bulletins/sexualidentityuk/2019 (accessed on 31 January 2022).

Office for National Statistics (ONS) (2021d) *Population Estimates.* Available at: www.ons.gov.uk/peoplepopulationandcommunity/populationandmigration/populationestimates (https://www.who.int/publications/journals/bulletin).

Office for National Statistics (ONS) (2021e) *National Life Tables – Life Expectancy in the UK: 2018 To 2020.* Available at: www.ons.gov.uk/peoplepopulationandcommunity/birthsdeathsandmarriages/lifeexpectancies/bulletins/nationallifetablesunitedkingdom/2018to2020 (accessed 4 June 2022).

Office for National Statistics (ONS) (2022a) *Coronavirus (COVID-19) Latest Insights.* Available at: www.ons.gov.uk/peoplepopulationandcommunity/healthandsocialcare/conditionsanddiseases/articles/coronaviruscovid19/latestinsights (accessed 8 February 2021).

Office for National Statistics (ONS) (2022b) *Population Estimates for the UK, England, Wales, Scotland and Northern Ireland: Mid-2021.* Available at: www.ons.gov.uk/peoplepopulationandcommunity/populationandmigration/populationestimates/bulletins/annualmidyearpopulationestimates/latest (accessed 11 February 2023).

Office for National Statistics (ONS) (2022c) R*eligion, England and Wales: Census 2021.* Available at: www.ons.gov.uk/peoplepopulationandcommunity/culturalidentity/religion/bulletins/religionenglandandwales/census2021 (accessed 11 February 2023).

Officer, A and de la Fuente-Núñez, V (2018) A global campaign to combat ageism. *Bulletin of the World Health Organization,* 96, 295. Available at: www.who.int/publications/journals/bulletin (accessed 7 August 2022).

O'Leary, L, Hughes-McCormack, L, Dunn, K, and Cooper, SA (2018) Early death and causes of death of people with Down syndrome: a systematic review. *Journal of Applied Research in Intellectual Disabilities,* 31(5), 687–708.

Oman, D and Thoresen, CE (2005) Do religion and spirituality influence health? In RF Paloutzian and CL Park (eds), *Handbook of the Psychology of Religion and Spirituality.* New York: Guilford Press.

Oozageer Gunowa, N, Hutchinson, M, Brooke, J, and Jackson, D (2018) Pressure injuries in people with darker skin tones: a literature review. *Journal of Clinical Nursing,* 27 (17–18): 3266–75.

Papadopoulos, I (2006) *Transcultural Health and Social Care: Development of Culturally Competent Practitioners.* Edinburgh: Churchill Livingstone.

Papadopoulos, I (2014) *The Papadopoulos Model for Developing Culturally Competent Compassion in Healthcare Professionals.* Available at: www.youtube.com/watch?v=zjKzO94TevA (accessed 3 February 2019).

Papadopoulos, I (2018) *Culturally Competent Compassion: A Guide for Healthcare Students and Practitioners.* London: Routledge.

Papadopoulos, I and Pezella, A (2015) A snapshot review of culturally competent compassion as addressed in selected mental health textbooks for undergraduate nursing students. *Journal of Compassionate Healthcare*, 2(3). Available at: https://jcompassionatehc. biomedcentral.com/track/pdf/10.1186/s40639-015-0012-5 (accessed 21 October 2019).

Papadopoulos, I, Tilki, M, and Taylor, G (1998) *Transcultural Care: A Guide for Health Care Professionals*. Dinton: Quay Publications.

Parliament UK (2019) *What We Know about Inequalities Facing Gypsy, Roma and Traveller Communities*. Available at: https://publications.parliament.uk/pa/cm201719/cmselect/ cmwomeq/360/report-files/36005.htm (accessed 19 September 2019).

Paul Victor, CG, and Treschuk, JV (2020) Critical literature review on the definition clarity of the concept of faith, religion, and spirituality. *Journal of Holistic Nursing*, 38(1): 107–13.

Pavord, E and Donnelly, E (2015) *Communication and Interpersonal Skills*. Banbury: Lantern.

Peate, I (2016) Transgender equality. *British Journal of Nursing*, 25(5): 239.

Pentaris, P (2018) The marginalization of religion in end of life care: signs of microaggression? *International Journal of Human Rights in Healthcare*, 11(2): 116–28.

Perez-Bret, E, Altisent, R, and Rocafort, J (2016) Definition of compassion in healthcare: a systematic literature review. *International Journal of Palliative Nursing*, 22(12): 599–606.

Pesut, B (2016) There be dragons: effects of unexplored religion on nurses' competence in spiritual care. *Nursing Inquiry*, 23(3): 191–9.

Phillips, C (2021) How COVID-19 has exacerbated LGBTQ+ health inequalities. *BMJ*, 372: m4828. Available at: https://doi.org/10.1136/bmj.m4828

Phillips, G, Lifford, K, Edwards, A, Poolman, M, and Joseph-Williams, N (2019) Do published patient decision aids for end-of-life care address patients' decision-making needs? A systematic review and critical appraisal. *Palliative Medicine*, 33(8): 985–1002.

Price, B (2017) Improving nurses' level of reflection. *Nursing Standard*, 32(1): 52–61.

Prins, H, Backer-Hoist, T, Francis, E, et al. (eds) (1993) *Report of the Committee of Inquiry into the Death in Broadmoor Hospital of Orville Blackwood and a Review of the Deaths of Two Other Afro-Caribbean Patients: Big, Black and Dangerous?* London: Special Hospitals Service Authority.

Public Health England (PHE) (2014) *Protecting Your Child against Flu: Information for Parents – Flu Immunisation in England*. Available at: https://assets.publishing.service. gov.uk/government/uploads/system/uploads/attachment_data/file/714954/PHE_ Protecting_Child_Flu_DL_leaflet.pdf (accessed 12 August 2018).

Public Health England (PHE) (2015) *Improving Health Literacy to Reduce Health Inequalities*. Available at: https://assets.publishing.service.gov.uk/government/uploads/system/ uploads/attachment_data/file/460709/4a_Health_Literacy-Full.pdf (accessed 26 April 2018).

Public Health England (PHE) (2017) *Tackling Tuberculosis in Under-Served Populations: A Resource for TB Control Boards and Their Partners.* Available at: www.gov.uk/government/publications/tackling-tuberculosis-in-under-served-populations (accessed 21 October 2019).

Public Health England (PHE) (2019) *PHE Strategy 2020 to 2025.* Available at: www.gov.uk/government/publications/phe-strategy-2020-to-2025 (accessed 8 February 2022).

Public Health England (PHE) (2020a) *Health Inequalities: Type 2 Diabetes.* Available at: https://fingertips.phe.org.uk/documents/Health%20Inequalities_Type2_diabetes.pdf (accessed 16 February 2023).

Public Health England (PHE) (2020b) *COVID-19: Understanding the Impact on BAME Communities.* Available at: www.gov.uk/government/publications/covid-19-understanding-the-impact-on-bame-communities (accessed 11 October 2022).

Public Health England (PHE) (2021) *Care Continuity Between Midwifery And Health Visiting Services: Principles For Practice.* Available at: www.gov.uk/government/publications/commissioning-of-public-health-services-for-children/care-continuity-between-midwifery-and-health-visiting-services-principles-for-practice (accessed 10 February 2021).

Purnell, L (2016) Are we really measuring cultural competence? *Nursing Science Quarterly,* 29(2): 124–7.

Qassem, T, Bebbington, P, Spiers, N, McManus, S, Jenkins, R, and Dein, S (2015) Prevalence of psychosis in black ethnic minorities in Britain: analysis based on three national surveys. *Social Psychiatry and Psychiatric Epidemiology,* 50(7): 1057–64.

Race Disparity Unit (2022) *Why We No Longer Use the Term 'Bame' in Government.* Available at: https://equalities.blog.gov.uk/2022/04/07/why-we-no-longer-use-the-term-bame-in-government/ (accessed 11 October 22).

Ramezani, M, Ahmadi, F, Mohammadi, E, and Kazemnejad, A (2014) Spiritual care in nursing: a concept analysis. *International Nursing Review,* 61(2): 211–19.

Rasheed, SP, Younas, A, and Sundus, A (2019) Self-awareness in nursing: A scoping review. *Journal of Clinical Nursing,* 28(5–6): 762–74.

Razai, MS, Chaudhry, UA, Doerholt, K, Bauld, L, and Majeed, A (2021) COVID-19 vaccination hesitancy. *BMJ,* 373.

Read, S, Heslop, P, Turner, S, Mason-Angelow, V, Tilbury, N, Miles, C, and Hatton, C (2018) Disabled people's experiences of accessing reasonable adjustments in hospitals: a qualitative study. *BMC Health Services Research,* 18(1): 1–10.

Rethink mental illness (2021) *Black, Asian and Minority Ethnic (BAME) Mental Health Fact Sheet.* Available at: www.rethink.org/advice-and-information/living-with-mental-illness/wellbeing-physical-health/black-asian-and-minority-ethnic-mental-health/ (accessed 11 October 22).

Richards, C and Barrett, J (2020a) 'Introduction to Gender Diversity' in C Richards and J Barrett (eds), *Trans and Non-Binary Gender Healthcare.* Available at: www.researchgate.net/publication/343744864_Introduction_to_Gender_Diversity (accessed 16 February 2023).

Richards, C and Barrett, J (2020b) 'Assessment' in C Richards and J Barrett (eds) *Trans and Non-Binary Gender Healthcare.* Available at: www.researchgate.net/publication/343744864_Introduction_to_Gender_Diversity (accessed 16 February 2023).

Richardson, B (2017) *Clinical Skills for Nursing Practice.* London: Routledge.

Richman, LS and Hatzenbuehler, ML (2014) A multilevel analysis of stigma and health: implications for research and policy. *Health and Wellbeing,* 1(1): 213–21.

Rickard, W and Donkin, A (2018) *A Fair, Supportive Society: Summary Report.* London: Institute of Health Equity, UCL.

Robertshaw, L, Dhesi, S, and Jones, LL (2017) Challenges and facilitators for health professionals providing primary healthcare for refugees and asylum seekers in high-income countries: A systematic review and thematic synthesis of qualitative research. *BMJ Open, 2017* (7): e015981. doi: 10.1136/bmjopen-2017-015981 (accessed 7 August 2022).

Robinson, F (2019) Caring for LGBT patients in the NHS. *BMJ,* 366: l5374.

Roper, N, Logan, W, and Tierney, AJ (2002) *The Roper–Logan–Tierney Model of Nursing: Based on Activities of Living* (3rd edn). London: Elsevier.

Rose, S, Hartnett, J, and Pillai, S (2021) Healthcare workers' emotions, perceived stressors and coping mechanisms during the COVID-19 pandemic. *PLOS ONE,* 16(7): e0254252. Available at: https://doi.org/10.1371/journal.pone.0254252

Rosmarin, DH, Kaufman, C C, Ford, SF, Keshava, P, Drury, M, Minns, S, Marmarosh, C, Chowdhury, A, and Sacchet, MD.(2022) The neuroscience of spirituality, religion, and mental health: a systematic review and synthesis. *Journal of Psychiatric Research,* 156: 100–113.

Rostosky, SS, Richardson, MT, McCurry, SK, and Riggle, ED (2021) LGBTQ individuals' lived experiences of hypervigilance. *Psychology of Sexual Orientation and Gender Diversity.* Available at: https://doi.org/10.1037/sgd0000474

Royal College of Nursing (RCN) (2010) *Principles of Nursing Practice.* Available at: www.rcn.org.uk/professional-development/principles-of-nursing-practice (accessed 10 August 2018).

Royal College of Nursing (RCN) (2011) *Spiritual Survey 2010.* Available at: www.rcn.org.uk/professional-development/publications/pub-003861 (accessed 13 August 2019).

Royal College of Nursing (RCN) (2016) *Caring for Lesbian, Gay, Bisexual or Trans Clients or Patients: Guide for Nurses and Health Care Support Workers on Next of Kin Issues.* Available at: www.rcn.org.uk/professional-development/publications/pub-005592 (accessed 28 September 2019).

Royal College of Nursing (RCN) (2017) *The Needs of People with Learning Disabilities: What Pre-Registration Nurses Should Know.* Available at: www.rcn.org.uk/professional-development/publications/pub-005769 (accessed 9 December 2019).

Royal College of Nursing (RCN) (2019) *Principles of Nursing Practice Videos.* Available at: rcn.org.uk (accessed 10 June 2022).

Royal College of Physicians (RCP) (2020) *COVID-19 and Mitigating Impact on Health Inequalities.* London: RCP.

Russell, C (2022) Meeting the moment: Bioethics in the time of Black Lives Matter. *The American Journal of Bioethics,* 22(3): 9–21.

Ryan, T (2022) Facilitators of person and relationship-centred care in nursing. *Nursing Open*, 9(2): 892–9.

Saini, A (2020) Stereotype threat. *The Lancet*, 395 (10237): 1604–5.

Sanford, M and Michon, NJ (2019) Buddhist chaplaincy. In *Oxford Research Encyclopedia of Religion*. Available at: https://doi.org/10.1093/acrefore%2F9780199340378.013.641

Sangar, M and Howe, J (2021) How discourses of sharam (shame) and mental health influence the help-seeking behaviours of British born girls of South Asian heritage. *Educational Psychology in Practice*, 37(4): 343–61.

Scadding, J and Sweeney, S (2018) *Digital Exclusion in Gypsy and Roma Travellers in the United Kingdom*. Available at: www.gypsy-traveller.org/wp-content/uploads/2018/09/Digital-Inclusion-in-Gypsy-and-Traveller-communities-FINAL-1.pdf (accessed 4 November 2018).

Scally, G (2021) *England's New Office for Health Improvement and Disparities*. London: British Medical Journal Publishing Group.

Schultz, PL and Baker, J (2017) Teaching strategies to increase nursing student acceptance and management of unconscious bias. *Journal of Nursing Education*, 56(11): 692–6.

Scope (2021) Disability facts and figures. Available at: www.scope.org.uk/media/disability-facts-figures/ (accessed 31 January 2022).

Scottish Learning Disabilities Observatory (2021) *Life Expectancy and Mortality*. Available at: www.sldo.ac.uk/our-research/life-expectancy-and-mortality/ (accessed 29 May 2022).

Seewoodhary, J (2021) Black Lives Matter: tackling racial and ethnic inequalities in diabetes health care. *Practical Diabetes*, 38(3): 26–30.

Setta, SM and Shemie, SD (2015) An explanation and analysis of how world religions formulate their ethical decisions on withdrawing treatment and determining death. *Philosophy, Ethics, and Humanities in Medicine*, 10(1): 6.

Shelter (2017) *More Than 300,000 People in Britain Homeless Today*. Available at: https://england.shelter.org.uk/media/press_releases/articles/more_than_300,000_people_in_britain_homeless_today (accessed 3 September 2019).

Shen, Z (2015) Cultural competence models and cultural competence assessments instruments in nursing: A literature review. *Journal of Transcultural Nursing*, 26(3): 308–21.

Sibiya, MN (2018) Effective communication in nursing. *Nursing*, 19: 20–34.

Simonovich, SD, Spurlark, RS, Badowski, D, Krawczyk, S, Soco, C, Ponder, TN, … and Tariman, JD (2021) Examining effective communication in nursing practice during COVID-19: A large-scale qualitative study. *International Nursing Review*, 68(4): 512–23.

Smith, S (2021) What's in a word? Rephrasing and refreshing and reframing disability. In N Brown (2021) *Lived Experiences of Ableism in Academia: Strategies for Inclusion in Higher Education*. Bristol: Policy Press.

Snowden, A (2021) What did chaplains do during the Covid Pandemic? An international survey. *Journal of Pastoral Care & Counseling*, 75(1 (supplement)): 6–16. Available at: https://doi.org/10.1177/1542305021992039

Solomos, J (2003) *Race and Racism in Britain* (3rd edn). New York: Macmillan International Higher Education.

Sommers, MS (2011) Color awareness: a must for patient assessment. *American Nurse Today*, 6(1): 6.

Sovacool, BK and Del Rio, DDF (2022) 'We're not dead yet!': Extreme energy and transport poverty, perpetual peripheralization, and spatial justice among Gypsies and Travellers in Northern Ireland. *Renewable and Sustainable Energy Reviews*, 160: 112262.

Spritzer, J (2003) *Caring for Jewish Patients.* Oxford: Radcliffe Publishing.

Srivastava, R (2003) *The Healthcare's Professional's Guide to Clinical Cultural Competence.* Canada: Mosby.

Starnino, VR (2016) Conceptualizing spirituality and religion for mental health practice: perspectives of consumers with serious mental illness. *Families in Society*, 97 (4): 295–304.

Stonewall (2018) *LGBT in Britain Health Report.* Available at: www.stonewall.org.uk/system/files/lgbt_in_britain_health.pdf (Accessed 10 January 22).

Sullivan, R (2014) A 5-year retrospective study of descriptors associated with identification of stage I and suspected deep tissue pressure ulcers in persons with darkly pigmented skin. *Wounds: A Compendium of Clinical Research and Practice*, 26(12): 351–9.

Tabassum, H (2022) *Sociology of Change and Development.* New Delhi: KK Publications.

Taylor, B and Hinks, J (2021) What field? Where? Bringing Gypsy, Roma and Traveller history into view. *Cultural and Social History*, 18(5): 629–60.

Terrence Higgins Trust (2019) *Equitable Access to PrEP Now.* Available at: www.aidsmap.com/news/jan-2019/six-innovative-models-prep-services (accessed 10 January 2022).

Tervalon, M and Murray-García, J (1998) Cultural humility versus cultural competence: A critical distinction in defining physician training outcomes in multicultural education. *Journal of Health Care for the Poor and Underserved*, 9: 117–25. *Project MUSE.* doi:10.1353/hpu.2010.0233 (accessed 14 November 2022).

The Albert Kennedy Trust (2021) *The LGBTQ+ Youth Homelessness Report.* Available at: www.akt.org.uk/report (accessed 10 November 22).

The Kings Fund (2015) Long-term conditions and multi-morbidity. Available at: www.kingsfund.org.uk/projects/time-think-differently/trends-disease-and-disability-long-term-conditions-multi-morbidity (accessed 16 February 2023).

The Kings Fund (2020) *Our Work On Health Inequalities and Access to Care for Different Groups in Society.* Available at: www.kingsfund.org.uk/topics/health-inequalities (accessed 8 February 2022).

The Kings Fund (2021) *The Health of People From Ethnic Minority Groups in England.* Available at: www.kingsfund.org.uk/publications/health-people-ethnic-minority-groups-england#Diabetes (accessed 10 January 2022).

Thelwall, M and Thelwall, S (2021) Twitter during COVID-19: George Floyd opening a space to address systematic and institutionalized racism? Available at: http://dx.doi.org/10.2139/ssrn.3764867

Thomas, R (2020) CORONAVIRUS 'Unprecedented' number of DNR orders for learning disabilities patients. *Health Service Journal.* Available at: hsj.co.uk (accessed 10 November 2022).

Timmins, F and Caldeira, S (2017a) Assessing the spiritual needs of patients. *Nursing Standard*, 31(29): 47–53.

Timmins, F and Caldeira, S (2017b) Understanding spirituality and spiritual care in nursing. *Nursing Standard*, 31(22): 50–7.

Tran, L, Wong, C, Leung, J, and Lam, J (2008) *Community Engagement Project: The National Institute for Mental Health in England Community Engagement Programme 20067/08. Report of the Community Led Research Project Focussing on the Mental Health Service Needs of Chinese Elders in Westminster, Kensington & Chelsea and Brent.* London: Chinese National Healthy Living Centre.

Tuffrey-Wijne, I, Giatras, N, Goulding, L, Abraham, E, Fenwick, L, Edwards, C et al. (2013) *Identifying the Factors Affecting the Implementation of Strategies to Promote a Safer Environment for Patients with Learning Disabilities in NHS Hospitals: A Mixed Methods Study.* Available at: www.journalslibrary.nihr.ac.uk/hsdr/hsdr01130/#/abstract (accessed 29 April 2018).

Tuffrey-Wijne, I, McLaughlin, D, Curfs, L, Dusart, A, Hoenger, C, McEnhill, L et al. (2016) Defining consensus norms for palliative care of people with intellectual disabilities in Europe, using Delphi methods: a White Paper from the European Association of Palliative Care. *Palliative Medicine*, 30(5): 446–55.

Turner, N, Hastings, JF, and Neighbors, HW (2018) Mental health care treatment seeking among African Americans and Caribbean blacks: what is the role of religiosity/spirituality? *Aging & Mental Health*, 23(7): 905–11.

Tyrer, F, Morriss, R, Kiani, R, Gangadharan, SK, Kundaje, H, and Rutherford, MJ (2022) Health needs and their relationship with life expectancy in people with and without intellectual disabilities in England. *International Journal of Environmental Research and Public Health*, 19: 6602. Available at: https://doi.org/10.3390/ijerph19116602

UKHSA (2021) *Tuberculosis in England: 2020.* London UKHSA. Available at: https://assets.publishing.service.gov.uk/government/uploads/system/uploads/attachment_data/file/1030165/TB_annual-report-2021.pdf (accessed 11 February 2022).

UK Parliament (2019) *Tackling Inequalities Faced by Gypsy, Roma and Traveller Communities.* Available at: https://publications.parliament.uk/pa/cm201719/cmselect/cmwomeq/360/full-report.html (accessed 12 February 2023).

UN Convention on the Rights of the Child (UNCRC) (1990). Available at: www.savethechildren.org.uk/content/dam/gb/reports/humanitarian/uncrc19-summary2.pdf (accessed 16 February 2023).

UNHCR (UK) (n.d.) UNHCR – What is a refugee? Available at: www.unhcr.org/what-is-a-refugee.html (accessed 7 August 2022).

United Kingdom Government (2021) *Guidance The NHS Constitution for England Updated January 2021.* Available at: www.gov.uk/government/publications/the-nhs-constitution-for-england (accessed 10 June 2022).

University of Bristol (2018) *The Learning Disabilities Mortality Review (LeDeR) Programme: Annual Report 2017.* Available at: www.bristol.ac.uk/media-library/sites/sps/leder/leder_annual_report_2016-2017.pdf (accessed 5 October 2019).

University of Bristol (2021) *The Learning Disability Review (LeDeR) Programme. Annual Report 2020.* Available at: www.england.nhs.uk/wp-content/uploads/2021/06/LeDeR-bristol-annual-report-2020.pdf (accessed 3 June 2022).

University of Warwick (n.d.) *People's History of the NHS.* Available at: https://warwick.ac.uk/fac/arts/history/chm/outreach/peoplesnhs/ (accessed 23 November 2022).

van Os, J (2012) Psychotic experiences: disadvantaged and different from the norm. *British Journal of Psychiatry*, 201: 258–9.

van Vliet, M, Jong, MC, and Jong, M (2018). A mind–body skills course among nursing and medical students: a pathway for an improved perception of self and the surrounding world. *Global Qualitative Nursing Research*, 5: 2333393618805340.

Venkatasalu, MR (2017) Let him not be alone: perspectives of older British South Asian Minority Ethnic patients on dying in acute hospitals. *International Journal of Palliative Nursing*, 23(9): 432–9.

Vos, T, Lim, SS, Abbafati, C, Abbas, KM, Abbasi, M, Abbasifard, M, Abbasi-Kangevari, M, Abbastabar, H, Abd-Allah, F, and Abdelalim, A 2020. Global burden of 369 diseases and injuries in 204 countries and territories, 1990–2019: a systematic analysis for the Global Burden of Disease Study 2019, *The Lancet*, 396: 1204–1222.

Waldron, IR (2019) Archetypes of Black womanhood: Implications for mental health, coping, and help-seeking. In *Culture, Diversity and Mental Health-Enhancing Clinical Practice* (pp. 21–38). Cham: Springer.

Wareham, J (2021) *Pandemic's Detrimental Impact On U.K. LGBTQ Community Revealed In New Research.* Available at: www.forbes.com/sites/jamiewareham/2021/11/09/pandemics-detrimental-impact-on-uk-lgbtq-community-revealed-in-new-research/ (accessed 10 January 2022).

Watson, J (1988) Nursing: human science and human care. A theory of nursing. *National Nursing League Publications*, 15–2236: 1–104.

Watson, J (2008) *Nursing: The Philosophy and Science of Caring* (rev. ed.). Boulder: University Press of Colorado.

Weerasinghe, S (2012) Inequalities in visible minority immigrant women's healthcare accessibility. *Ethnicity and Inequalities in Health and Social Care*, 5(1): 18–28.

Welch, K (2022) *Effective Communication for Nursing Associates.* London: SAGE.

Welsh Government (2018) *Learning Disability: Improving Lives Programme.* Available at: https://gweddill.gov.wales/docs/dhss/publications/learning-disability-improving-lives-programme.pdf (accessed 28 September 2019).

Werner, S and Shulman, C (2015) Does type of disability make a difference in affiliate stigma among family caregivers of individuals with autism, intellectual disability or physical disability? *Journal of Intellectual Disability Research*, 59(3): 272–83.

Wessendorf, S (2014) *Commonplace Diversity: Social Relations in a Super-Diverse Context*. New York: Springer.

White, K (2002) *An Introduction to the Sociology of Health and Illness*. Available at: www.nacro.org.uk/data/files/prevalence-patterns-and-possibilities1051.pdf (accessed 2 May 2017).

Wilkins, A, Mailoo, VJ, and Kularatne, U (2010) Care of the older person: a Buddhist perspective. *Nursing and Residential Care*, 12(6): 295–7.

Williams, A (2021) Health inequalities among LGBTQ+ communities. *The British Student Doctor Journal*, 5(2): 88–94.

Williamson, EJ, Mcdonald, HI, Bhaskaran, K, Walker, AJ, Bacon, S, Davy, S, Schultze, A, Tomlinson, L, Bates, C, and Ramsay, M (2021) Risks of COVID-19 hospital admission and death for people with learning disability: Population based cohort study using the OpenSAFELY platform. *BMJ*, 374.

Williamson, M and Harrison, L (2010) Providing culturally appropriate care: a literature review. *International Journal of Nursing Studies*, 47: 761–9.

Wilson, B, Woollands, A, and Barrett, D (2018) *Care Planning: A Guide for Nurses* (3rd edn). Harlow: Pearson Education.

Wood, JT (2004) *Communication Theories in Action: An Introduction* (3rd edn). Belmont: Wadsworth.

World Health Organization (WHO) (1948) *WHO Constitution*. Geneva: WHO. Available at: www.who.int/about/who-we-are/constitution (accessed 29 September 2019).

World Health Organization (WHO) (2008a) *A Global Approach to Health Equity*. Geneva: WHO. Available at: www.who.int/social_determinants/final_report/csdh_finalreport_2008_part1.pdf (accessed 3 September 2019).

World Health Organization (WHO) (2008b) *Closing the Gap in a Generation: Health Equity through Action on the Social Determinants of Health*. Geneva: WHO. Available at: http://apps.who.int/iris/bitstream/handle/10665/43943/9789241563703_eng.pdf?sequence=1 (accessed 29 August 2019).

World Health Organization (WHO) (2008c) *Social Determinants of Health: Key Concepts*. Geneva: WHO. Available at: www.who.int/social_determinants/thecommission/finalreport/key_concepts/en/ (accessed 6 October 2019).

World Health Organization (WHO) (2011) *Behind the 'Glasgow Effect'*. Geneva: WHO. Available at: www.who.int/bulletin/volumes/89/10/11-021011/en/ (accessed 29 August 2019).

World Health Organization (WHO) (2013) *Health Literacy: The Solid Facts*. Geneva: WHO. Available at: www.euro.who.int/__data/assets/pdf_file/0008/190655/e96854.pdf (accessed 28 April 2018).

World Health Organization (WHO) (2018) *Noncommunicable Diseases (NCD) Country Profile.* Geneva: WHO. Available at: www.who.int/nmh/countries/gbr_en.pdf (accessed 10 January 2022).

World Health Organization (WHO) (2020) *The Impact of the COVID-19 Pandemic on Noncommunicable Disease Resources and Services: Results of a Rapid Assessment.* Geneva: WHO.

World Health Organization (WHO) (2021) Global report on ageism. Geneva: WHO. Available at: Global report on ageism (who.int) (accessed 7 August 2022).

World Health Organization (WHO) (2022a) *The Global Health Observatory: HIV/AIDS.* Geneva: WHO. Available at: www.who.int/data/gho/data/themes/hiv-aids (accessed 10 February 2022).

World Health Organization (WHO) (2022b) *Tuberculosis: Key Facts.* Geneva: WHO. Available at: www.who.int/news-room/fact-sheets/detail/tuberculosis (accessed 11 January 2022).

World Health Organization (WHO) (2022c) Disability. Geneva: WHO. Available at: www.who.int/health-topics/disability#tab=tab_1 (accessed 4 June 2022).

World Health Organization (WHO) (n.d.) *Health Topics: Health Policy.* Geneva: WHO. Available at: www.who.int/topics/health_policy/en/ (accessed 4 September 2019).

Wylie, K, Knudson, G, Khan, SI, Bonierbale, M, Watanyusakul, S, and Baral, S (2016) Serving transgender people: clinical care considerations and service delivery models in transgender health. *The Lancet*, 388 (10042): 401–41.

Younis, T (2021) The muddle of institutional racism in mental health [Commentary]. *Sociology of Health and Illness*, 43(8): 1831–9.

Zegers, C and Auron, M (2022) Addressing the challenges of cross-cultural communication. *Medical Clinics*, 106(4): 577–88.

# Index